Paula Horan

# Abundance
# Through

# *Reiki*

### Universal Life Force Energy
### As Expression Of The Truth That You Are
### The 42-Day Program To Absolute Fulfillment

MOTILAL BANARSIDASS PUBLISHERS
PRIVATE LIMITED

*First Indian Edition: Delhi, 1997*
*Reprint: Delhi, 1997*

© 1990. Windpfred Verlagsgesellschaft mbH,
Aitrang, Germany.
All Rights Reserved.

Published by arrangement with Lotus Light Publications,
P.O. Box 325, Twin Lakes, WI 53181, USA

ISBN: 81-208-1476-2 ( Cloth)
ISBN: 81-208-1477-0 ( Paper)

*Also available at:*

**MOTILAL BANARSIDASS**
41 U.A. Bungalow Road, Jawahar Nagar, Delhi 110 007
8 Mahalaxmi Chamber, Warden Road, Mumbai 400 026
120 Royapettah High Road, Mylapore, Chennai 600 004
Sanas Plaza, Subhash Nagar, Pune 411 002
16 St. Mark's Road, Bangalore 560 001
8 Camac Street, Calcutta 700 017
Ashok Rajpath, Patna 800 004
Chowk, Varanasi 221 001

PRINTED IN INDIA

BY JAINENDRA PRAKASH JAIN AT SHRI JAINENDRA PRESS,
A-45 NARAINA INDUSTRIAL AREA, PHASE 1, NEW DELHI 110028
AND PUBLISHED BY NARENDRA PRAKASH JAIN FOR-
MOTILAL BANARSIDASS PUBLISHERS PRIVATE LIMITED,
BUNGALOW ROAD, DELHI 110 007

*This book is dedicated to*
*H.W.L. Poonja*
*who has opened my heart*
*to the brilliance of Self beyond mind*

# Table of Contents

# Acknowledgments

Almost seven years have passed since I wrote *Empowerment Through Reiki*. At that point I had the feeling that I had said all I would ever want to say about Reiki. Much has happened since then, which has opened me to a greater depth of knowledge, and, more profoundly a deeper sense of Being. I am very grateful for having had the opportunity to practice Reiki and to teach it all around the world.

For the last few years my connection to my spiritual teacher H.W.L. Poonja has been the greatest source of inspiration to me, and thus it is with deep gratitude that I have dedicated this book to him. His unconditional love and open heart have revealed true Self to me—the Source of Universal Life Force Energy.

I am also thankful to my Indian partners Upen and Anjana Chokshi, because in some sense they prompted me to write *Abundance Through Reiki*. They are both successful and deeply commited Reiki masters and encouraged me to explore the correspondence between true Self and Universal Life Force Energy and to share the results of my exploration with others.

I also want to thank my father Robert Horan for once again offering me a quiet space in his home to commit my ideas to paper. I thank my husband, Matthias Dehne, for all his help, inspiration and cooperation. He has been with me all the way, beginning with the first discussions of the ideas for this book and throughout the process of writing and rewriting several drafts of the manuscript.

My first book *Empowerment Through Reiki* has been translated into twelve languages and is welcomed in many countries as a basic reference on the subject of Reiki. I wish to thank my publishers Wolfgang and Monika Jünemann for their enthusiasm and tireless efforts in getting it out there.

And to all of you who have gifted me with your unique piece of the "abundance pie", I offer my heartfelt gratitude and wish you well on your journey into greater abundance.

## Song of Abundance

*Every moment*
*the One Moment*
*when being here*
*is just a drop*
*and carried to the sea*

*every moment*
*the One Moment*
*when doing stops*
*forever done*
*fruit growing on the tree*

*every moment*
*the One Moment*
*when heart is love*
*and soothed in love*
*is never known to cease*

Narayan

# Introduction

*If Reiki is Universal Life Force Energy, and you and I are*
*the same Universal Life Force Energy, it stands to reason*
*that the Usui method of natural healing*
*is an effortless process*
*of applying to oneself and others*
*more of what we essentially already are.*

*Abundance Through Reiki* introduces you in a very practical manner to the connection between Universal Life Force Energy and true Self, awakening you to the deep knowledge of abundance which is your true nature. Concrete examples from my own and the experience of others show you how through applying Universal Life Force Energy you can liberate yourself from being emotionally hooked and blocked. In addition, the texts and commentaries to the exercises point the way to fulfillment through self-inquiry. By listening and sensing deep into yourself you will discover that this fulfillment is not different from your true or Core Self. In other words: Reiki, the Usui method of natural healing, will eventually guide you to the experience that you yourself *are* Reiki or Universal Life Force Energy.

Reiki has flourished all over the world in the past few years. There are more and more practitioners who have been initiated into all three Degrees. Much has happened since my first book *Empowerment Through Reiki* came out in 1989, and even more has been written about Universal Life Force Energy in papers, magazines and books. Most of these publications focus on physical and/or psychological healing. It is easy to understand why this approach has been emphasized, since perfect health is the symbol of wholeness that we all wish to achieve in our lives.

However, in the more than eight years of my own practice as a Reiki master I have experienced and taught Reiki in a slightly different fashion, namely with a childlike openness and as the totality of being—as an energy incomprehensible to the intellect which flows though everything, transforming all realms of life, enriching them with an abundance of new perceptions and experiences. Reiki is an art of living, and at the deepest level, Reiki is ONENESS.

The more complete our surrender is to the Universal Life Force Energy we are at heart the more open we become to its transformative power. The more we delve into it, the more mysterious it seems to be. It becomes increasingly difficult to explain. Fortunately with Reiki, this ceases to be a problem, because during the course of years of practice we also tend to lose our addiction to intellectual explanations. Instead, we begin to live in the moment. We experience life at gut level, with our immediate and spontaneous feelings, no longer in our heads and with the thoughts that divide and separate.

This book has essentially two parts. The first three chapters describe some of the qualities and peculiarities of Reiki. I also relate my own experiences with Reiki to illustrate how it has been a path to absolute fulfillment for me. Beginning with chapter 4, the second part explains the 42-day program to absolute fulfillment, gives handy hints and describes the positive changes which occur after completing the program.

The examples and exercises are designed to help you open up to the abundance and fulfillment, and to the unimaginable richness which is at the heart of who you truly are. As the focus of my presentation is the subject of abundance, I do not go into depth with a lot of the other aspects of Universal Life Force Energy. If you wish to learn more about the attunements, hand positions during treatment, and the healing aspects of Universal Life Force Energy, I suggest my first book *Empowerment Through Reiki* as I give an in depth presentation on all of these subjects. Better yet, participation in a Reiki course is my best advice, after careful selection of a master.

A Reiki course is not a prerequisite for the successful completion of the 42-day program to absolute fulfillment. You don't have to apply Reiki for good results on your path to abundance. However, Reiki can *support* you on this path. If you wish to integrate Reiki into the processes of the 42-day program, you have to be able to practice Reiki, which means you need at least the First Degree attunements. In any event, actual practice is the only effective approach to Reiki. It may be fun and inspiring to read about Reiki, but in terms of actual results, only the loving and regular application of Reiki will prove effective. Ideally this application happens in the form of whole body treatments or through spontaneously putting your hands wherever your body seems to need Universal Life Force Energy. Special positions for special indications are rarely needed.

Thus, *Abundance Through Reiki* is for all who seek to experience deep fulfillment through the direct experience of true Self, and for all of you Reiki practitioners who live Reiki as an all-encompassing path enriching your life with an unlimited Source of Universal Life Force Energy.

My intention in this book is to provide the reader with the opportunity to shed some light on the personal patterns of lack. I aim to bring them into your awareness so that you can eventually dissolve them. A belief in or feeling of lack restricts your development and comes in many different forms, such as lack of love, lack of understanding, lack of joy or whatever lack you encounter in your life. You can equate this lack to a mirror, reflecting back to you where and how far you have alienated yourself from true Self—from your own Source of aliveness, vitality and abundance. I also intend to demonstrate the all-pervasive and wholesome nature of Reiki. Reiki can only have positive healing effects, because Reiki is reclaimed by you through the attunements of a qualified master from a level of reality which dissolves all polarities in the Oneness of Universal Life Force Energy. Reiki is not subject to the polarities of "good" or "bad" or any such pair of opposites, which is why Reiki can help liberate us from our attachment to duality or polarized consciousness and lead us to the Ocean of Consciousness itself.

Through the experiences of the 42-day program you may realize that you come from this same source—that *you are* indeed the very same Source. The commentaries and exercises will help you to experience this reality. They will assist you in opening to the abundance of true Self, so that eventually you will experience that everything is coming to you and flowing through you, because in the eternal now of your Source, you *are* everything. You will discontinue living as a small and restricted ego with all its resistances and desires. Rather you will melt into the all-encompassing I AM which allows all positive and negative experiences to happen and flow through, without attachment, without getting hooked.

Throughout the text some words may appear on occasion in capitals. This is to indicate that they point to the *whole* of reality which transcends and encompasses all polarities. These key words are not put in capitals in all instances, only occasionally to prod your awareness. They suggest that you can neither *achieve* nor *accomplish* true Self or Universal Life Force Energy, because you always have been, you always are and you always will be true Self. Thus you do not need additional exercises or "advanced practices" which are presumably designed "to boost" Universal Life Force Energy (how can you boost what already is all-encompassing, all-pervasive and ever-present?). What you may need is an occasional impetus or impulse to become more fully aware so that you are able to *consciously feel* and appreciate your own deep truth. In this sense Grand Master *Phyllis Furumoto* (the only grand master in the direct line of *Hawayo Takata*) has stated: "The Master gives the student nothing he or she does not already have, nor does the Master take away anything that is not already absent." True Self can neither boost nor diminish true Self.

As mentioned in the acknowledgments, this book is dedicated to my master *H. W.L. Poonja.* He has shown me beyond the slightest shred of doubt that there is nothing to realize, that everything is *here,* that everything happens *now,* and that we only have to open our eyes for one split second to truly see and receive the abundance of life and love that we already *are.* Some forms of expression are taken from his and the great tradition of Ramana Maharshi. They are inspired by the Indian philosophy of *advaita* (non-duality) which states that nothing exists, only true Self. In this respect, they correspond with all other great spiritual traditions of the world which, at heart, focus on "Knowing One-Self". At the heart of all spiritual traditions is the intention to support people so they can directly experience and live who they *truly* are, beyond the conditioning and limitations of the small "self" or personality. By increasingly opening us to the flowing presence of Universal Life Force energy, Reiki is one of these great traditions.

Thus, the processes of the 42-day program are not techniques that enhance Reiki. Rather, they should be considered stepping stones for deepening your conscious awareness. They actually trigger concrete results as you can see from the experiences shared in chapter 5 and other chapters. By diligently practicing the two 21-day plans of the 42-day program you will dissolve many fears and open to a more joyful sense of being. You will also appreciate more fully what it truly means to be alive.

Before you get to this point, you will have the opportunity to make peace with all the aspects of yourself which bring up your resistance. The program will guide you and provide a means to help you deeply feel and dissolve many of the attachments which keep you in lack. Once this process is complete, you can focus on the abundance inherent in your life—and on the joy inherent in it.

Laced throughout the entire book is the important realization that abundance must be approached from an understanding that the "I" or ego can of itself do nothing, although it hypnotizes us in the illusion that it does a lot. It is the ability to instead turn your attention inward to true Self or Universal Spirit that enables and empowers a consistent flow of abundance in your life. Positive affirmations will work to a certain degree, but only if spoken from true Self. If they are stated from ego or false "self", its negative shadow aspect will eventually rise to the surface and create havoc with any progress made by these same affirmations. We need to address the ingrained negative beliefs first, or at least (and preferably) simultaneously with the positive, to experience any real success. Throughout the chapters that follow I hope to help you do just that. May this book inspire for you the deep inner peace which flows when you are truly coming from Divine Source.

Chapter 1

# What Is Reiki?

Reiki is the Japanese word for Universal Life Energy. To most people just gaining familiarity with Reiki, it is generally known as an ancient healing art rediscovered about a hundred years ago by Dr. Mikao Usui. As this is primarily a book on abundance, I will dwell not so much on the healing aspects of Reiki but recommend in addition, my previous book *Empowerment Through Reiki* which covers such information in detail, and better yet, participation in an actual Reiki course to gain first hand experience.

Before continuing into the subject of Reiki and abundance, it seems appropriate to include at least a short synopsis of Reiki and a description of how this transformative energy is used as a healing tool. As stated above, Reiki is the Japanese word for Universal Life Energy. When the "Rei" and "Ki" are broken down into their component parts, the *Kanji* (Japanese Alphabet) definition for Reiki is: Transcendental Spirit, Mysterious Power, Essence. In my previous book, I stated that we all have Reiki energy (Universal Life Force Energy) for it is our birthright. To be precise one could actually say that we *are* Reiki or Universal Life Force Energy, for it is the very "stuff" we are made of. Even science now recognizes the fact that so called solid objects are just densely vibrating energy, that, in fact, there is no solid matter. Hermetic science also states that "all is energy".

Hermetic – Impervious to liquids or gasses
Impervious – not permitting passage of fluids, light
rays etc – impenetrable –

15

*Cloudbanks dissolve*
*soil smells of summer rain*
*droplets on emerald leaves*
*still lingering*
*under the great mysterious sun*
*shining forth from heart*

Narayan

In the Usui system of Natural Healing, a person attending a Reiki course receives what are called attunements or initiations that help open them up to receiving more of this energy through the laying on of hands. There are various stages of energy amplification, which is why Reiki is divided into three degrees. During Dr. Usui's time, students would travel with him, slowly becoming initiated over a period of years into the various levels of energy through the attunement process until they could also become teachers. During this century, the division of attunements into degrees has made it easier to disseminate the various stages of initiation. Before completing each successive step or degree it is good to allow oneself an adequate period of time to adjust to a higher vibratory frequency by allowing the sloughing off of old patterns which occur with the daily practice of Reiki.It is also important to allow enough time to master the skills of each succeeding level before proceeding to the next. Optimally, one should use First Degree at least three months before proceeding to Second Degree (if not longer), and then wait a minimum of three years after Second Degree before considering Third Degree (the master level). Quite a few people in recent years, excited by the amazing results of Reiki, have rushed through the three degrees, cheating themselves out of a very rich process. Reiki, like a fine wine, is to be savored and experienced slowly, not "slugged down", so that you miss its essence.

16

Another story I share with my students regarding the foolishness of rushing life is the example of the modern young couple who fall in love (or lust as the case may be), jump in bed, make mad passionate love, and then are confronted with the embar"ass"ing fact that they haven't even made friends yet. Most modern Westerners who have been through a few relationships have learned the importance of getting to know each other first; to develop a deep intimate relationship, so that later sex becomes an expression of that depth, not a hindrance the day after. Reiki is much the same; in my years of training Reiki masters (Third Degree level) it is clear to me, that the ones who have waited the longest, who have used Reiki and developed their own processes with it, are richer and happier for it. They also had less chance of falling into the ego trap of some who have rushed through and actually been temporarily set back in their development as a result.

When savored and used over time, Reiki becomes much more than a simple healing method which abates our unpleasant physical symptoms for the time being, until we foolishly take up our bad habits again. It actually helps old negative behavior patterns fall away; such as overeating, smoking, overworking etc., so that we no longer create illness or attract freak accidents. In short, over time, Reiki accelerates our process toward spiritual maturity.

As I established earlier, we all have Reiki energy, as in actuality, we are that—Universal Life Force Energy. What makes Reiki different from other healing methods, is the attunement (also known as initiation) process which the student experiences in a Reiki course. Anyone can lay their hands on another person and help accelerate the healing process by transferring electro-magnetic energy. A person who has been through the process of Reiki attunements however, has experienced an ancient technology for fine tuning the physical and etheric bodies to a higher vibratory frequency without effort.

During the attunement process, a Reiki master acts as a

mirror to help the student attune her- or himself to the Reiki energy. This energy acts in such a way that it creates an open "channel" for cosmic or universal energy. Through this channel Reiki then flows in through the top of the student's head, down through the body and out through the hands, during treatments. In addition, the vibratory rate of the body is amplified, triggering a 21-day cleansing process which occurs as a result of negative patterns and blocks being sloughed off due to the quickening of a person's energy pattern. The attunements are very precise and can only be transmitted by a Reiki master who has been trained in the Usui method. It is good to seek out several masters and find one with whom you feel a mutual bond or resonance.

Attunements affect each person differently, depending on your vibratory frequency when you first receive them. In other words, if you have spent time doing work to expand your awareness, and have steadily increased your vibratory level, the attunements will provide a very quick quantum leap to an even greater opening. To someone just beginning self-inquiry, there is also a quantum leap, but the expansion of energy will be relative to the level you start with. Thus you always receive only what you can handle. One of the great benefits of Reiki is that, even after the quantum leap which is initiated by the attunements, you can still continue to increase your vibratory frequency by treating yourself or others daily, whenever possible.

First Degree attunements seem to have a powerful effect on opening up the physical body so that it can then accept (channel) greater quantities of Reiki energy. The four attunements of First Degree effect the etheric or energy body as well, but seem to have their greatest impact on the grosser physical body at this initial level. Once you are attuned to Reiki energy, you never lose it. Even if you don't use it over a period of years, it will be there for you. The channel however, becomes stronger with use.

The Second Degree attunements provide aother "quantum leap" in vibratory frequency. The three symbols which are taught in Second Degree, and used for absentee healing, also become activated at this point. At the Second Degree level, the attunement seems to have a much greater effect on the etheric or energy body. As all the chakras or energy centers are contained in the etheric body, often a lot of energy is released. Soon after the Second Degree attunement process, and especially during the 21-day cleansing process, people often feel a considerable amount of energy in the root chakra, because the survival and sexual centers, and other areas where they have been blocked become stimulated. One of the more obvious effects of the Second Degree attunement is also the heightening of one's intuitive abilities as the "third eye" or ajna chakra also seems to get stimulated. My own ability to perceive the etheric body occurred right after Second Degree.. What I have discovered over the years is, that each student has his or her own forte in this realm; some have more of a tendency towards clairaudience, some to clairsentience, some to clairvoyance. Whatever each person's natural ability is, it often gets heightened after Second Degree. With further practice at the Second Degree level, a further letting go seems to happen along with a resulting deeper sense of peace.

*Whatever inner worlds I choose to explore*
*or how subtle and etheric my sensations may become*
*no matter how far over time and space I travel*
  *in order to heal -*
*I AM going nowhere and nothing is coming to me*
*in this silent celebration of unity*

Narayan

Clairvoyance — ability to see or know things, not perceptible to normal human senses

19

The Third Degree attunement is used to initiate a master; it again seems to amplify the vibratory level and activates the master symbol so it may be used to help others empower themselves. This is an important point, because it is essential for people to realize that it is their choice to receive an attunement. A Reiki master holds no lordly power over his or her students. A Reiki master is simply a person who has chosen to take the next step into mastership by accepting a greater level of responsibility for his or her life. He or she openly accepts the effects of causes which are self-created. By accepting this responsibility, the Reiki master is empowered to use specific processes to assist others in further empowering themselves. The attunement process of Reiki is really exceptional, in that it enables you to get in touch with your true essence. We tend to sense this essence or Core Self at times in our lives, when we are in a heightened state of awareness. Reiki can provide the boost to help you develop that sense of awareness, and with a daily practice of self-treatments, enable this awareness to grow.

An important point to understand about Reiki is that it is never sent. Thus there is no "doing" involved. It is always drawn through the channel. Even at the Second Degree level, which enables you to transmit the energy across time and space, it is drawn. The symbols enable you to create a "bridge" to another, over which the energy can be drawn. Because of this you can never give a person too much Reiki, including yourself. For example, if I lay my hands on you to do a treatment, your body will naturally draw the appropriate amounts of energy it needs, and to the proper places. I am never drained in this process, as I too am treated as I give a treatment. According to studies at Stanford the energy seems to enter at the area of the crown chakra (at the top of the head), and also passes through the heart area to my hands and then to your body. I am never drained in the process, as a certain amount of energy passing through, is actually absorbed by me, enabling me to receive my own treatment simultaneously. Also at the same time, the receiver does not take on any of my negative energy or blocks, as Reiki passes through a purified channel in my body opened by the attunement process.

One of the greatest benefits of Reiki is the possibility of self-treatment. Once you are attuned, you need only have the intention to do Reiki on yourself or another, and the energy is immediately drawn through. Self-treatment is a very effective technique for relaxation and stress release. It amplifies the Life Force Energy in the body which then helps to create balance in the physical and etheric bodies. Treating oneself also helps to release withheld emotions and energy blocks.

Each person draws in just the right amount of Reiki that he or she needs to release, activate or transform the energy in the physical and etheric bodies. Reiki not only effects change in the chemical structure of the body by helping to regenerate organs and rebuild bone and tissue, it also creates balance at the mental level. The harmony and balance which happens as a result of Reiki treatments, happens of its own accord and is not effected by the wishes or desires for any particular result of the practitioner. All outcomes are different for every treatment, the *healee* being the determining factor of the net result.

Reiki is not a religion or dogma as it holds no creed or doctrine. It is a very ancient science or healing art hidden for thousands of years until Dr. Usui rediscovered it. As it is also not a belief system, no mental preparation or direction is needed to receive a treatment, only a simple desire to receive and accept the energy. Also from the standpoint of the practitioner, since it is not a belief system, and no rituals are needed, once the intention is clear to start a treatment, it will always be activated. The key is that the healee be open to receiving the energy. A recipient of Reiki need not believe in it, he or she only has to have a sincere willingness to try it and most of all, some sort of investment in his or her own healing process. For example, it is essential that a person ask for a treatment and not be pressured to accept one. The simple act of asking for

21

help is in itself a reaching out which infers the person is willing to receive. At times, an exchange of energy is also important and should be considered, as this shows a willingness to take responsibility for one's own health, and frees the person of obligation to you. Eventually the person should be encouraged to take a Reiki class, so he or she can begin taking full responsibility for his or her own health and wholeness. Reiki is truly a spiritual discipline, as realizing the importance of taking responsibility for all that you create in your life is indeed one of the keys of Reiki. Reiki shouldn't end after the First or Second Degree class. Each person must take responsibility to continue self-treatments. You are indeed your own master. Only you determine your own rate of development, by *your* level of commitment to Self. The exhilaration which is experienced as each level of awareness is unveiled over time, makes it all worthwhile.

From the above we can see some of the unique aspects of Reiki. Like other healing methods, it helps each individual find balance and harmony in Body, Mind, and Spirit. Reiki is truly a gift to oneself. It enables you to slowly drop your attachment or identification as a doer and to come from a source of being. No longer attached to the doer you are free to simply be.

# Chapter 2

# Reiki and Abundance

If Reiki is Universal Life Force Energy, and you and I are that same Universal Life Force Energy, it stands to reason that the Usui method of natural healing is an effortless process of applying to oneself or others, more of what we essentially already are. When you consider this statement deeply, the implications are quite profound. Mystics have realized forever that individuals are actually the very Energy of the Universe personified.

Finally, in our day and age, this knowledge is becoming part of popular culture. However, what has not happened so far in great numbers, is the actual internalization of this knowledge. People readily accept the idea of quantum physics, that everything is energy; that there is no real solid matter; but has this insight changed anything in their lives? Most people would answer in the negative. It has not brought them a new car, new or better relationships, better health, or any of the other things they desire. All the new information on energy has just not hit home yet.

What most people don't realize, is that energy is the most essential commodity in our lives, and I am not referring to the gas in your car or your electric bill. If who we are is energy, and all solid matter is energy, then all our cars, homes, money and even relationships are also forms of energy.

When we arrive on this playground of dense vibration, we have already made the decision to experience restriction. The role we play is predetermined, so what is left but the game of seeking to transcend it all by trying on the beliefs that get us back to "GO" fastest? Life is similar to a big monopoly game, where instead of collecting a lot of things (although that can be a large part of it), we collect a lot of experiences, which help us learn how to expand our energy fields. Due to this expansion we are enabled to move right through the feeling of separateness caused by the restriction of matter, and restore our true state of union. This game would not be so complicated if we only had to deal with things and people. What becomes our greatest hindrance in the game, is our attachment to all our beliefs and judgments (the same ones we were only supposed to try on).

All the thoughts which form the background of our everyday lives, are formed or filtered through the judgments and beliefs we have become attached to, and which in turn each have their own vibratory frequency. Positive thoughts fill our consciousness with high vibratory energy; they help us expand our energy outward which is essential to the "game". Negative thoughts or judgments have a very dense energy; they contract us inward energetically, leaving us with a very small sphere of influence. Other people in the game will feel repelled by this energy, and when you are in a "down cycle" you will feel yourself suddenly surrounded by others of the same dense vibration. Extra will and energy is needed to pull out of this cycle.

If you examine history, it is one long sad tale after another of people competing for energy by fighting over territory, religious beliefs, money, wealth, relationships etc. The participants at some point got so used to receiving energy from one another on this dense playground of earthly matter, that when some became dense themselves, and could no longer channel the finer energy directly from Source (because they had become identified with their negative beliefs or judgments), the rest of the players also followed suit, began to absorb the same dense energy and thus bought into the idea of lack.

We have been involved in this cycle of false dependency for quite some time now, learning and playing out all of its various forms. Essentially what has happened during this long, arduous cycle is, that people have forgotten that *they are the very energy of life itself*—the very energy they so determinably chase after outside themselves in all its various outward forms. Each one of us already has direct access to all the energy we want; we only have to turn our awareness inward to true Self which is common to us all, and instantly it is taken care of. Everything we could ever imagine and more becomes accessible. It sounds easy, and actually it is, but due to the fact that we are totally delirious, absolutely and completely identified with mass consciousness, it seems downright impossible.

The players in the game have become identified with the various thoughts of who they are, the variety of things they just "have to have", and the things they "have to do", that they have lost track of the fact that their thoughts are not their consciousness, are not indeed who they are. The thoughts we "choose" or actually get hypnotized by are what feed our consciousness, and it is the type of thoughts and emotions we focus on that shape it.

Consciousness is in truth both your awareness, and your understanding of everything you have ever experienced. Until you turn inward to the Universal Power which is individualized as you, for all your needs, you will remain affected by mass consciousness, or what Carl Jung called the "collective unconscious" of man (the sum total of all human experiences).

For most human beings, consciousness is the vehicle through which Universal Life Force Energy flows, to create in the world of matter the exact reflection of whatever each individual's thoughts or beliefs are. At this stage, people are for the most part operating robotically, totally unconscious of the fact that they are in no way "in control".

Most people experience in the outer world of matter an exact duplicate of their belief systems, which includes whatever cultural beliefs are ingrained unconsciously. For those who are still "asleep", consciousness functions as the vessel through which creative energy flows into form and experience. For such a person it may seem, as if life "is doing it to you", for this same consciousness works as an effect to produce a like effect. In other words you tend to magnetize toward you whatever your mind is consumed with.

It is only later when you gain a broader view and drop your attachment to your various beliefs and identities, that a true sense of mastery arises and you begin to cooperate with Source, with true or Core Self. You no longer feel separate or at odds with the world as duality consciousness begins to loose its grip. This process in myself has been supported with the practice of Reiki.

If Reiki is the application of more of the "stuff" I am made of, it certainly follows that over time my energy field will naturally expand (the more I do self-treatment). As consciousness is included in this package, it will also expand, taking me beyond my normal narrow scope of getting hooked on thoughts into a more relaxed "all seeing" kind of awareness. As my awareness expands, with this awareness, my range of possibilities in the outer world also expands. I gradually develop a larger sphere of influence and an abundance of everything I am now open to, naturally flows toward me.

*With all my cells*
*relishing the waters of Life*
*from formless hands of light*
*ecstasy flows through*
*to unlock the treasure chest inside*

Narayan

Reiki is truly one of the most powerful and yet simple tools available in our time, to help everyone open to greater realms of possibility in all areas of life. To reap the real benefits of Reiki, one must first be open to receiving the flow of this abundant Life Force Energy.

The story of Dr. Mikao Usui's experience in the beggars' quarter of Kyoto illustrates this same need to be open to the vast supply which is available to us, and also expresses our need to give back to the universe in some form, for that which we have received. The importance of an exchange of energy, a constant flow of give and take, became clear to him after seven years with the beggars. When Dr. Usui first became empowered to perform the miracle healings he had sought for so long, his first decision was to move to the beggars' quarter in true "Christian" style and serve the poor. He decided to use his powerful channel of Life Force Energy to help heal the beggars so that they could become responsible citizens, and to help enable them to hold jobs to support themselves. What he discovered seven years later, was that many returned after having experienced a taste of life on the outside, and decided that they didn't want the responsibility of caring for themselves.

In other words, much of his work had been unappreciated as there was no real openness to receiving what it was he had to share. By just "giving away" healings he had further impressed the beggar pattern in many of them. It began to dawn on him that people needed to give back for what they received, in order to fully appreciate what had been given. People needed an investment in their own healing or growth.

In addition, Usui realized that his own missionary zeal to "fix" the beggars was the root of his intense frustration at his failure to convert them to a so-called ordinary and responsible way of life. It became clear that he had been on a major "ego trip" in terms of deciding what was good or proper for anyone else. It also began to dawn on him that the great success of Christ's healings was not the fact that Christ was a great healer,

27

but it had been his very non-attachment to the results of the healings that made him such a success. Eventually Usui probably remembered that Christ took no credit for his healings, that indeed he had said: "By your own faith you are healed."

Finally, Dr. Usui realized that even though he himself had been graced with an extraordinary ability to channel Life Force Energy, it was the readiness in the other to *receive* the energy, that determined the true results. Also by having an attachment to the results of his own healing work he had created resistance in the other to receiving the full benefit of his assistance. His ego attachment to getting certain results had very likely blocked the ability of the other to receive.

It was now totally clear that in fact the final outcome rested entirely on the healee's total willingness (both conscious and unconscious) to receive the results of treatment; to actually draw energy in.

Usui thus discovered two very important factors: One that a person should ask for a healing (it is not the job of any healer to try and help where help is not wanted); and two, that there should be an exchange of energy for the healer's time (it is not right to keep someone feeling indebted for services rendered, thus the healee, by sharing energies in a variety of forms, frees himself of obligation).

After about seven years in the beggars' quarter, Usui left. He began a period of deep self-assessment, and while meditating on his next course of action, he received new information on how to use the symbols he had experienced seven years earlier during the powerful vision which had changed his life. He realized he could work with these symbols in a certain way to help others, who were now open to this energy, empower themselves. Dr. Usui devised a way to initiate and attune mankind to Reiki, so that each individual could choose to use it for him- or herself and also share it. From this point on, he began to work only with people who were willing to take full responsibility for their own life process. Whereas before he had tried to "do it all for others", he now began to teach the importance of responsibility for oneself, and most of all, the attitude of gratitude. He now used the symbols he had seen seven years earlier in his vision to attune people, so that they could take responsibility for their own well-being. By helping them amplify their energy, they could then take a bigger step toward their own mastership over "self" or ego, and in turn become more in tune with true Self, which is common to us all.

Previously Usui had placed too great an emphasis on the healing of the physical body. He now understood that the healing of the Spirit was every bit as important, and actually more so, as the root of physical problems were a result of mind being out of sync with reality. In truth, the causal factor of disease lies in the gross misunderstandings of most of humanity as to who we truly are. The painful separation most people experience energetically due to their beliefs that they are separate and not a part of the whole, manifests in a variety of forms. If I feel separate from my husband, wife, children, family, friends or co-workers; if I am angry and feel out of control in any situation; if I am worried about anything; all of these boil down to one fatal mistake: complete identification with an "I" separate from the whole, or separate from the vast sea of Universal Spirit of which I AM in truth very much a part.

To those who have never experienced a deep sense of oneness this may seem very abstract. In fact, as long as one is "stuck in one's head" it is virtually impossible to experience this unity, as the mind, so identified with an "I" manifesting as ego rather than true or Core Self, along with the accompanying restriction of a physical body in matter, keeps this sense of separation constantly in effect. It is this very "I" thought which takes over and interprets our sensory experience in such a way, that further amplifies this sense of separation from true Self.

For a person who finds it difficult to quiet the mind and get out of his or her head, Reiki becomes a powerful tool to relax and let go. With Reiki, physical complaints and symptoms disappear due to the quieting of the mind, as one's energy comes into balance. Most people after receiving Reiki several times, begin to fall asleep quickly during each succeeding treatment. This is a very good sign, as in fact it is only while asleep that the "I" thought finally disappears, and the average person comes in direct contact with true Self. During sleep the body has a much greater capacity to heal, as it is not fighting off the willful thoughts and reactive emotions connected to the "I" thought.

In order to maintain good health and a flow of abundance in one's life, we need to turn inward toward true Self. We need to transcend this sense of separation that leaves us feeling insecure, and begin to realize that the ego is not something we have to dissolve or fight or get rid of, but a tool created by the mind to help us operate in the world. The ego is indeed an illusory creation of mind, and as such, doesn't even really exist. To waste time fighting or resisting it, only makes it seem more "solid" or real, as resistance only gives it further energy and strength.

By consciously recognizing we are not ego, that we are a part of something far greater than it, and turning instead to true Self—the source of all that we are—we stand a chance of experiencing the Union we so urgently desire. Reiki adds great support to this intention, as it is not influenced by mind or ego. As an inherently "intelligent" energy, it goes directly where it is needed to create balance in body and spirit.

The more we use Reiki, the stronger our channel becomes for this flow of Universal Life Force Energy. As the energy flows, it eliminates the blocks which otherwise might cause illness or keep us from receiving the abundance which is truly ours. Reiki amplifies our creative energy, and as money is a symbol of our creative energy in the outer world, it stands to reason that Reiki also helps increase the flow of wealth both within and without.

An excellent example of the power Reiki evokes to increase creative energy is one of the first treatments I gave after receiving First Degree. It was to an artist friend in California who had been feeling very depressed because she hadn't been inspired for several months with any fresh, new ideas. The day after her treatment she called me up all excited, wanting to know just what that "energy work" was, that I had used on her in addition to her regular massage treatment. She told me excitedly how relaxed she had felt when she got home; that she had taken a short nap, and when she woke up had started and then completed a whole new sketch. To top it off, she had even been up the whole night painting at least a third of the canvas. When I told her it was called Reiki, an ancient healing art designed to dissolve blocks and create balance in body, mind and spirit, she enthusiastically signed up for several more treatments. Eventually, she took a Reiki course herself and became a Reiki advocate in the art community. Since that time I have had similar responses to Reiki from artist friends all around the world.

I have used the previous example many times in my First Degree classes to emphasize to people that Reiki is for much more than just relieving physical pain and symptoms. It is a tool to help you open up in all areas of your life. It is there to help you energize your creativity, and to help you break down your blocks to both giving and receiving abundance. The physical and mental health Reiki evokes, and the physical healings which take place, are just an added benefit which occur due to the blocks in awareness which are melted away, thanks to its gentle but persistent effect on consciousness.

Another very important story about Reiki and abundance consciousness was related to both Fran Brown and Helen Haberly in their respective books on Hawayo Takata's life story. Takata was a Japanese American woman who brought Reiki to the West in the1930's. Her teacher Dr. Chujiro Hayashi was Dr. Usui's successor. Whereas Dr. Usui, who after leaving the beggars' quarter in Kyoto, traveled around Japan leading a very nomadic life while teaching Reiki, Dr. Hayashi instead centralized Reiki through his decision to open a clinic in Tokyo. It was here that Hawayo Takata first came, to receive treatments while on a visit from America. Inspired by her own miraculous cure after three months of treatment, she was determined to learn this powerful healing art. Initially, Hayashi was very closed to the idea of passing on this healing method to a "gaijin" or foreigner, but as luckily Takata had an influential friend, she was finally able to persuade him to train her. After a long apprenticeship when she devoted all her time to Reiki, she was finally ready to return home to Hawaii.

Before she left Japan, she had to ask Hayashi one last question which had been bothering her. During her year at the clinic and the times she had accompanied Hayashi on house calls, she had never come in contact with poor people; not even blue collar workers or laborers. She wondered if he refused to treat such people. At first Hayashi laughed, but with a knowing look he quickly responded that she had asked a very good question. He explained that indeed all the people who were drawn to him were upper class, even titled people who were intelligent, educated, and mostly wealthy. In actual fact they could afford the best doctors and hospitals, but having experienced these, they sought more than surgery and drugs. They had Reiki consciousness themselves, so they were attracted to him. The people who had not accessed this abundance or knowledge did not share the same understanding. When illness struck, instead they felt a need for shiny hospitals, doctors, nurses, and drugs. They sought relief in the outer world of effect. Hayashi explained to her that if called, he would go, no matter how poor they were, but as their beliefs were different, it was unlikely they would accept him or his drugless treatment. He suggested that when she became a full fledged practitioner, she would in all probability also find this to be true.

To a large degree what Hayashi conveyed to Takata in the 1930's is still very true today. For the most part the vast majority of people still seek a quick fix for their suffering in the outer world of effect. Although Reiki is far more available today than it was fifty years ago, many people still take Reiki classes initially with the same attitude they go to the doctor with. Like a pill which gives instant relief, they often hope Reiki will provide an instant cure after one treatment. Whereas I have been blessed with my own share of these instant miracle cures over the years, they are most often few and far between. It usually takes several days or weeks before the causal factor is dealt with and the cure is complete. Years of toxins collected in the body do not often disappear overnight.

What does seem to have changed since Hayashi's time and especially after World War II, is the education of the masses, especially in the Western world. Wealth became more evenly distributed in the 50's, 60's and 70's, and large numbers of people found more leisure time not only to pursue the outward pleasures of life, but also to seek inward for nourishment at a deeper level.

In the last ten years Reiki has become a world wide phenomenon. As we move into the 21st century in this day and age of accelerated growth and change, Universal Life Force Energy has become a necessity. It is as essential as food and water, as the very air we breath. No longer can we afford to stay in the consciousness of lack, fighting each other off to get our "piece of the pie", or competing for energy by fighting over territory, religious beliefs or wealth. This energy has always been there for us, we somehow just forgot how to access it.

The Usui method of natural healing is a practice which helps us regain that access so we no longer have to suffer lack. Reiki consciousness is abundance consciousness. As Phyllis Furumoto, Takata's granddaughter has stated: "In Reiki, you are given the gift of having your memory, and your innate power reawakened." From this state of wholeness and balance all things become possible. Abundance becomes a way of life.

*Separated for eons*
*or so it seems*
*I still remember YOU*
*the Force that I forget*
*I always AM*
*and in this moment of recognition*
*I AM reawakened*
*to Being undivided*

Narayan

Chapter 3

# Journey into Abundance

## The "Success" Model

Like many women of my generation who chose a life style devoted to career in the liberated 70's, I initially developed a very masculine style of moving through the world. For the most part, it didn't often seem that our mothers had enjoyed life as much as our fathers, so we chose the model which would most likely get us where we needed to go. Thus in the process of breaking free of too many generations of repressed women, many young women at the time, like myself, began to model themselves after the successful male. Basically in the *yang* or masculine way of doing things, you decide what it is you want, and whatever it takes, you go after it full force, which many of us did with great gusto.

During this period many women discovered that indeed, they had a very powerful animus or male aspect and could do just as well or better than many of their male counterparts. Women now had the opportunity to experience the male side of things, and during this process we also discovered that the "grass is not always greener on the other side". What we began to notice was, the *yang* or masculine way of doing things often involved a lot of struggle. As the focus always tends to be on "getting" or acquiring something outside of yourself, duality consciousness becomes even more accentuated making you feel increasingly separate from the whole. The masculine way of doing places a lot of emphasis on gaining satisfaction in the outer world. A lot of focus is put on acquiring possessions and because in much of past history survival often depended on

35

stockpiling things, one could easily surmise that fulfillment must be found in the accumulation of material wealth.

To succeed one had to know how to act effectively, accruing lots of knowledge the yang way. Since the time of Descartes until very recently, little emphasis has been placed on the more feminine, intuitive side of knowledge. In the old masculine ruled world which is now shifting to a more balanced feminine/masculine one, rationalization and logic held sway.

Previously, woman's intuition was not to be trusted, which resulted in great struggle, as everyone evolved into going the route of figuring things out the hard way, when often all you needed was to tune in to the right answer already there inside of you. Murphy's law, which states that "if something can go wrong it will go wrong" exemplifies the struggle inherent in the masculine mentality. Trust in the universe, or in one's own inner knowing is not cultivated; on the contrary, too much emphasis is placed on backing one's decisions on "expert" outside advice. Basically, you are most often cajoled into towing the line by your family, friends, co-workers, and society in general, as they have a vested interest in having you stick around.

So, the current and fading "success" model is one that alienates you from your source, as it does not bring you the all-encompassing abundance that can be yours in any moment. If on the other hand you opt for abundance and open to its flow, success will come to you of its own accord. You will have managed to blend intuition and reason, and both the feminine way of receptivity and the masculine way of applying oneself vigorously.

# The Struggle for Money

In the old success model, a lot of emphasis is placed on accumulating money or things, and there is often not a lot of joy in the process of acquiring it. With such an attitude you are doomed to struggle because you begin to think that money itself is important. You unconsciously begin to buy into the belief that money itself has actual value, and you lose sight of the fact *that money is only an effect*. In truth, true or Core-Self is the only one *real source* of the abundance you were born to enjoy. Money is only a symbol of energy exchange and as such it has no intrinsic value. The cost or value of things (including your labor) is purely an emotional decision, thus the sooner you disengage from your emotions about money, the better your chances are of attracting it.

Most of us have been brought up with a variety of negative teachings about money: "You've got to work hard for your money." "Life isn't easy." "Life is not all peaches and cream." "If I only had more money, I could do what I want." "Money is the root of all evil." "Rich people don't make their money honestly." And so forth. All of these and similar statements have been deeply ingrained in our subconscious, and our ego, due to its mission to help us survive in the world, takes them very seriously. If you believe you have to work hard for your money to survive, you can be sure your ego will make sure you do just that. On the other hand, if you are worried about what others think about you and you need their approval, you'll probably end up feeling guilty if you make "too much" money or more than the others in your circle.

Thus it can be seen, the ego is a major hindrance to any abundance plan. Even if you are overflowing with money, you probably harbor feelings about losing it. Essentially, as long as you are identified with ego and any of its "black and white" or polarized ideas about money, you are going to be afraid; even if you deny or try to ignore the feeling. The ego is always on guard for your security, and until you are in touch with Core Self and have developed a trust in the true source of your wealth, you are doomed to a life of uncertainty.

To find fulfillment one has to move away from either of the two extremes in life. On the masculine side, competition becomes a major focus, whether it be in business or struggling for resources, or recognition. Competition automatically implies that something is lacking—that there is not enough to go around -whether it be a lack of customers, a lack of money, or a lack of love. In truth there is always plenty of everything available. In business, even if there are many other companies similar to yours, you only have to use a little ingenuity to make yours stand out and endow it with your own special energy, to draw in a regular supply of customers.

In truth, there is no such thing as security in the physical world anyway as the human body is very fragile. Thus to waste precious hours of your life trying to support a total illusion of security is absolute folly. Only trust in true Self which is not subject to physical death will ever bring a sense of peace.

If you observe nature carefully, in terms of resources, there is actually more than enough food and money for everyone to be rich (there is only a major distribution problem), and as for love, this is the actual energy of the universe. Instead of chasing after love outside of ourselves, we need to get in touch with the fact that we already have a direct connection to an unlimited supply.

By tuning in to true or Core Self which is common to us all, we connect ourselves with this limitless reservoir of love energy. Love only seems lacking when we seek it outside of ourselves. It is true that people reflect it back to us, and we need love from others to feel nourished. In truth however, they are only responding to the love which is already flowing through us from the same source. Tuning into abundance is simply a process of letting go and letting love through you.

On the other side of the coin, the feminine approach to

38

fulfillment is simply to recognize what is already always there, and allow it to flow through. There is no longer anything to chase after or fight for. For most people of either sex, the trick to developing this very feminine ability to channel as well as enjoy abundance, rests in one's capacity to receive love.

*The very air I breathe*
*is given to me abundantly*
*the Life Force that makes my heart beat*
*is an offering to be renewed moment by moment*
*countless realizations of Truth*
*are presented in continous flow*
*ultimately*
*I surrender*
*and accept love's invitation*
*to boundless Life*

Narayan

Most people actually crave love, as we tend to resist the very thing we need the most. We resist love, because we have to open our hearts to receive it. This openness or vulnerability we need to cultivate in order to receive, threatens the protective wall that ego has built. The clutching neediness which results when we block love's flow, only acts to push it further away. Because of the terrible sense of separation that results, we then tend to put up even more blocks to protect our vulnerability, and our neediness increases once again.

To break this all too common pattern, you may initially have to muster a lot of courage. At some point we just have to take a leap of faith, break though our fear and begin to cultivate a long forgotten trust in the universe. Everything we need is already inside us, just waiting for us to shift our awareness and allow it to flow. To do this we have to drop the ego's attempts to control, which ultimately amounts to self-sabotage, and instead turn toward our own inner bastion of all knowledge and overflowing energy—Core Self.

## Fulfillment Through Balance

The ability to live from Core Self requires that a certain balance or harmony between the inner masculine and feminine be achieved, but as we have seen, in the West today, and in most of the world, the masculine aspect—the rational, active, aggressive power of the mind, is dominant. What we can do now to counteract this tendency, is begin to cultivate the more feminine qualities such as intuition, and a greater sensitivity and awareness. The more passive qualities of the feminine allow us to just *be*, rather than always being focused on doing.

Ultimately what is needed is a balance between the two. Most men and successful career women who have ignored their feminine needs in favor of a more masculine mode of operation will find tremendous fulfillment by developing the ability to do all the necessary activities of life, while coming from a more feminine, calm state of being.

Also women who have lived out a more feminine role, yet who have bought into the "superior" male model, may now need to open up and learn how to actively pursue what it is they want, and draw on their masculine energy. This is similar to the East, where the feminine aspect, the intuitive, passive, sympathetic power of the mind is dominant, therefore there may be a need there to take on a more active "doing" role in the world. The future of the planet depends on the marriage of these two minds; the conscious and the unconscious, the rational and the intuitive, the active and the passive.

To go beyond success and finally experience self-fulfillment, we need to utilize both the masculine ways of doing and the feminine ways of being. Together the two bring us into a state of unity where the natural order of abundance and self-fulfillment can occur.

## The Attitude of Gratitude

The most simple and powerful way to develop an abundance consciousness is to cultivate the attitude of gratitude. One of the five Reiki principles, it has also been one of the most powerful tools in my life, helping me to move quickly from a consciousness of lack to an abundance of love, health, friendship, knowledge and wealth. Very soon after I came in contact with Reiki, many wonderful changes occurred in my life. The list of things and variety of experiences would take several volumes to relate.

At the time, I was studying and teaching several different healing modalities, some of which had no tangible references in reality as we know it. I had a strong desire to understand what I was observing, and somehow after my Second Degree, certain abilities I had never dreamed of, opened up and I was then able to experience another level of reality.

The wonder and gratitude I felt at the time for this incredible expansion seemed to have no boundaries. I found myself constantly saying "Thank You" to my teachers (both inner and outer) and to the universe in general. It seemed the more I gave thanks, the more I was flooded with more experiences, more challenges, and more of the knowledge I had sought for so long. All the verification I needed was immediately at my fingertips.

"Chance" encounters with strangers provided just the right information I needed to complete some project. The more I gave thanks, the more I experienced a synchronicity of events which brought all the puzzle pieces of my life together. For moments in time when I would express this gratitude, a sense

41

of peace and fulfillment would literally flood my body with a warm tingly glow. It was at these times that I realized I wanted to live in this state all of the time. It became very clear that by concentrating on gratitude, I was always focused on the state of "have". By being thankful for what I have, the universe just kept rewarding me with more.

It also became clear to me at this time, that all the riches I was receiving, would not necessarily be considered riches by another, but because they were the riches I sought and felt gratitude for, they continued to flow. By feeling rich and in a flow of abundance, I just continued to experience more riches. At times, my old conditioned patterns would rise up in reaction to some unexpected circumstance. This would shut off the flow, and then I'd have to make a concerted effort to get myself back on the track of appreciation. I sometimes used the old adage: "Fake it till you make it." Soon I was back in the attitude of gratitude. I learned very quickly that to stay too long in the attitude of "not having" would bring me only more of the same: the state of not having.

At times, when some of my shadow aspects would come up, and I just couldn't resist whining or complaining, I'd allow them just 15 minutes to "have it all out", and then I'd resume the attitude of gratitude. It began to dawn on me how really important it is, to be in just as much gratitude for the so-called negative experiences in one's life, as it is for the positive. Somehow this overall attitude of gratitude I'd cultivated, opened my eyes to the benefits of some of the more challenging and unpleasant experiences I sometimes found myself in. These were all important lessons along the way, and even if I couldn't always make sense of them, I relegated some of the more unpleasant circumstances to past bad karma "coming back to get me", and I could now at least be thankful that it was finally over. If my karma snuck up and it happened again, this was just a test to make sure I'd really completed the lesson.

In retrospect when I look back on my life so far, I realize

that somehow, no matter how traumatic things have been at times, I've always managed to take it in stride and look for the positive aspect in every experience. I've learned that it is not so important what happens to you, as it is, how you *interpret* what happens to you. If I interpret something in a negative way and as a result begin to resist it, I will then attract more of the same. If on the other hand I can look into the causal factors of experience and see for example that my mother didn't ignore me when I was six because she didn't love me, but because she was busy with two other children, or my husband is grouchy today not because I've done something wrong, but because he is overworked at the moment, I won't take life so personally.

The way you interpret experience has everything to do with how you feel about yourself. If I love myself and acknowledge the fact that I am a vehicle for universal abundance in all its various forms, chances are I'm going to experience that abundance. If on the other hand I feel like a victim of circumstances, that people are not to be trusted, and that I'm never going to get out of this situation, the likelihood is, the universe in all its infinite generosity will prove those very beliefs true. You will indeed fall victim time and time again; people will prove themselves over and over again to be totally untrustworthy, and you will never get out of this situation!

If however one day, you decide to try on a new belief; if you somehow begin to evoke new feelings about yourself, you stand a strong chance of experiencing a totally *different* reality. The average person has no idea how powerful beliefs really are in terms of their effect on our outer experience, for if we all did, we'd have a very different world. One good thing about these so-called "negative" experiences though, is that they attract more of the same over and over again, *until you finally wake up* one day and notice your pattern. As a result you then move to a new level of existence and no longer keep magnetizing it over again.

A simple way to shift into a new positive reality is, to regularly treat yourself with Reiki and cultivate the attitude of gratitude; to cultivate the feeling of love for everyone you meet, everything you do, and most of all, for your presence here on this earth. If I keep my thoughts on the great and wonderful things that I would like to do, then, as the days go by, I will find myself unconsciously seizing upon the opportunities that are required for the fulfillment of my desires. If I picture in my mind the capable, experienced person I desire to be, the thought I hold will constantly be transforming me into that particular individual.

Hermetic science states: "All is mind; all is vibration." I have found in my experience, if I maintain a positive mental attitude and focus on the good in every situation, my life takes on the identical positive vibration, and I then attract more of the same. As Friar Elbertus once stated: "To think rightly is to create. All things come through desire, and every sincere prayer is answered. We become like that on which our hearts are fixed. Carry your chin in, and the crown of your head high. We are gods in the chrysalis."

## Abundance of Health

The secret to a healthy body is a healthy mind, free of the vibrations of stress, and unconscious, repressed negative thoughts and their resulting emotions. To free yourself and welcome an abundance of health in your life, what is called for, is to raise your vibratory level. We are living at a crucial turning point in the earth's evolution. Everything is speeded up due to the incredibly powerful love vibration which is sweeping the planet.

When this love energy come in contact with any of the dense or "thick" vibrations of anger, sadness, fear or rage, stored in our bodies, a cleansing process is initiated. This cleansing process may manifest itself as the common cold when you have not allowed yourself to express your grief or sadness. Also, cancerous tumors are often a result of anger or deep rage turned inward on oneself. Another example is arthritis, which is usually due to an intense withholding (control issues) begun in childhood and carried over into adulthood. If you look at the causal factor of disease, it can generally be traced to blocked feelings accompanied by toxic waste buildup.

All dis-ease in the body/mind has a denied feeling behind it. If a feeling is denied for lifetimes it may manifest as an illness to the point where we may have to experience it our whole life in order to clear it or bring it into balance. On the other hand, there are many examples of miracle cures which have defied medical understanding, where AIDS or cancer patients thought to be on their death bed, were completely healed. This simply means that the causal factor for the illness has been cleared on a very deep level.

The very idea of getting in touch with unacceptable feelings may turn you off, but there are few alternatives if you wish to survive in this new level of energy. As the vibrations of the earth rise in frequency in line with the rest of the universe, you will need to feel your feelings fully in order to stay in balance with the rising vibrations of the world around you. All the thoughts you put out consciously or unconsciously in turn magnetize an exact repeat performance in your everyday experience. The same negative conditioning which keeps you feeling separate from true Self, is responsible for the stress, the upsets, all the illnesses and the grief that we draw to ourselves on a daily basis.

All our emotional upheavals are reactions to our conditioned thought patterns. What is called for, is to get in touch with the deeper feelings of love, and our very need for love, which lie underneath these emotional reactions. To do this we need to learn to dive right into the emotional feelings and experience them fully; energetically sense them fully so that they finally dissipate. In essence, we need to go right through them until we contact the love on the other side.

When you finally accept all your feelings, no matter how unpleasant, your life will take a tremendous shift into balance and harmony. In the *Core Empowerment Training* that I teach around the world we work on developing this very skill. It is so important to learn how to get out of your head and get back in touch with your feelings. It becomes much easier to stay healthy, as you no longer have a need to express your negative emotions through illness.

It is important to understand that different types of emotions each have a different rate of vibration. What we normally refer to as "negative" emotions are actually just a very dense version of "positive" emotions. They are uncomfortable, because they are so intense. Your own vibration which is magnetic, draws to you whatever it is your energy is doing at the time. A positive thought or emotion is like looking through a wide angle lens, you see the whole picture. The vibration is light and easy, so you have a greater perspective. The energy is very relaxed. Fear however, is like looking through the lens in a microscope. It is intensely focused. You thus end up putting more energy into fear in order to dissipate it than you would put into a positive thought. Because fear is so highly focused, when you resist it, your own energy ends up drawing to you the very experience or feeling that you fear the most, even if you are not aware of them.

The typical response when you are in denial of some feeling and are inadvertently put in touch with it, when someone mirrors it to you, is to build a thicker wall around it, so that you don't have to experience it. When you choose not to accept your feelings, unconsciously you end up magnetizing the very same denied feelings to you, so that eventually you have to experience them anyway. If they are still denied, they often develop into an illness. Occasionally you may even attract an accident to force you to finally face your feelings.

The only car accident I ever had occurred when I was under great stress, having made a terrible decision which went against my deeper knowing. Rather than waiting for such an abrasive wake-up call, it is much easier to embrace your feelings the first time round, as this quickly brings your energy into balance. Strong emotions then cease to have power over you, and you are freed, no longer giving your power away to these emotions or to a set of circumstances.

Finally, when dealing with illness, one important feeling you *can* cultivate, is love for your actual ailment or illness. I do not mean love in the way a hypochondriac loves illness, but to love it for the message it is giving you. What I have experienced with the various illnesses in my life, is that they have acted as a sort of temperature gage to show me where my thoughts or ideas were out of synchronization with reality. All emotions, positive or negative, are a reaction to thought. The true deeper feelings lie hidden underneath all of the surface emotions. If you can learn to love your illness and be thankful to the pain or discomfort for pointing out where you have been in denial, chances are it may quickly disappear.

Love energy will always reduce your resistance to your feelings dramatically. When your feelings can flow freely, vibrant health becomes possible. When you allow an abundance of love to flow through you, you will then live and share an abundance of health.

*When I see you with an open heart*
*my heart is opened further*
*into a unified field*
*where hate melts into love*
*and love is oneness*
*uncreated*

Narayan

# Abundance of Love

It is essential to tune into the love that is all around us if we are to receive the abundance which is truly ours. Unfortunately, most people are not in contact with this infinite supply of love. Instead we spend much of our time trying to please others. Most of us unconsciously, try to please our family, friends, and co-workers in order to barter for the love we so deeply crave, but will not acknowledge.

We seek recognition outside of ourselves which can never replace the love which is already there inside of us, just waiting for us to experience. This deep need for approval can be traced to the development of the ego, the illusory identity created by the mind, which we use to manipulate our way through the physical world. Because of our strong identification with the ego or personality, we have lost touch with who we already really are—a vehicle or vessel of Universal Life Force Energy. There is no need to seek approval, and thus love outside of ourselves, for we are composed of love energy itself.

If you are that very energy, you only have to wake up to that fact, to have it operate in your life. It all comes down to a simple switch in consciousness: a shift from a consciousness of lack (which is what you have been brainwashed with by the unconscious mass hypnosis of many egos having bought into lack for eons), to an awareness of the infinite being that you are. You are much more than all your thoughts, feelings and emotions, much more than all your ideas of who you are and your beliefs which filter your experience of reality. You are the very substance or energy of the universe itself, and therefore are already in direct contact with it. It is only your attachment to your beliefs about yourself and the world around you, which shroud your deep inner knowing and keep you from this realization.

The only way to break through this consciousness of lack is to surrender the ego (which is only a construction of your mind) to the greater Universal Life Force that is you. You don't have to fight your ego, or try to subdue it, or even wipe it out; you simply relegate it to its proper position. The ego is simply our landmap for moving through the world of physical form. It is there to help us survive, and thus it has picked up some peculiar habits along the way according to each persons conditioning and prior circumstances.

Whatever actions may have been appropriate for your survival when you were a child, are probably no longer necessary. However, the ego cannot know that. It is like a computer program, reacting to life robotically; doing what it deems is most applicable in the present circumstance, according to past experience. The problem is, it often blocks you from feeling what is appropriate in the present moment, through its preconceived notions of what worked best in the past, and may not necessarily pertain any longer. For example you may resist intimacy now by pushing others away, in effect shut them out, because as a five year old you did the same in order to protect your vulnerability (which was trampled upon time and again by insensitive parents or siblings). This proclivity of the ego to protect us, is the very essence of our need to be right.

At certain times we have needed to be right so that we could make the correct decision in order to survive. Nonetheless, in day to day relationships, this need to be right can become an insidious habit, which robs us of the intimacy we so deeply need in relationships and leads us into more pain and suffering. In order to make yourself right, most often you end up making someone else wrong, and as we all know no one likes to be made wrong. The end result is that you push the other person away and end up alone and feeling separate.

The tendency is to just keep on projecting the same insensitivity we experienced as children on the people we are in relationship with at the moment. We may blame them and make them wrong because we feel needy. Unconsciously they end up "obliging" us by actually acting out the same negative behavior patterns we have come to expect, even if this is *not* their natural proclivity.

This constant projection on the present of a past reality, is what binds us and keeps us reliving the same miserable patterns over and over again. We automatically assume others will treat us as we have come to expect and because we are attuned to a certain frequency of behavior, we usually attract the perfect person to act it out. An extreme example is the battered child who then attracts a mate later in life to reenact the same pattern. As children, we so desperately crave love and attention that we will even come to accept negative attention as an indication of love, if that is all that is offered.

What it comes down to, is that what we experience in life, is exactly what we have come to picture in our minds. If you change your mind and your expectations, your whole life changes. The people and situations you will attract, will be a direct reflection of your beliefs about yourself.

To counteract the pattern of constantly attracting what you don't need, due to old outmoded beliefs, there is a very simple solution. One of the most profound lessons I have learned in my life is simply to ask for what I need. After having played the role of the "independent" totally self-sufficient career women, it took me years before I could allow myself to become vulnerable enough to simply ask for what I need. Having played the teenage rebel role to the maximum in my early years, I continued the pattern by always being sure I could take care of myself. In all my relationships with men, I could never say "I need you". As far as I was concerned, to say such a thing would reveal a weakness I could not acknowledge at the time, and which would make me feel terribly vulnerable. As a result I went through several relationships which eventually all ended in a deadlock, as neither of us could ever commit or even admit that we needed one another.

This incredible need for love we all have, if left unacknowledged, leads to a terrible sense of neediness. If we allow ourselves to reach the level of neediness where we become desperate to find a partner simply to help assuage our hunger for love, we will find this very neediness sends any possible companion running. No one is attracted to a needy person, because a needy person has drained him- or herself of the ability to give, as well as to receive, on a very deep level. Only a rescuer type (who is just as needy) will be drawn in.

Whenever you come to a point where you allow yourself to feel your need, and openly express it to another, your need suddenly disappears. Paradoxically, the only way to transcend neediness, is to openly express that need—not resist it. Just like the pain which disappears when you put all your attention on it, neediness disappears when you allow yourself to feel the need.

It is helpful to consider that, at the deepest (or highest) level, we don't really need others because "others" are just different expressions of true Self. They only help mirror what we already are deep inside, for *they* are intrinsically *who we* already are. How can you need something that you already are? You were never separate to begin with! To help understand this truth which seems so confusing when you view it from the vantage point of a person with a "separate" body, it pays to look at how experience is processed by the mind.

Everything we experience actually happens entirely through the mind which is composed of all our thoughts and beliefs of how things are. We interpret all the circumstances in which we find ourselves with the mind. Thus, what we are really dealing with (our thoughts), is entirely unseen. Our experience of others is also only in our thoughts, because even though we may touch them physically, we interpret that touch in our minds. It follows easily from this, that the essence of who we are is entirely unseen—and completely limitless, as are all "others" we experience with the mind. True Self just presents itself time and again in a variety of forms, the body being just a denser vibration of all-mind, giving the illusion of being separate from "others".

51

The ego or persona, as the mind's vehicle for experience in the world, begins to identify with the body as a "self" separate from the whole. This identification as a separate "I", sets in motion a major downward spiral into matter. We hook into all the thoughts which justify us as a separate "self" and conclude that all others are just as separate.

The mind gets hooked on the ego, and the ego gets hooked on the body. Feeling terribly separate and alone and embroiled in the five senses, we hook onto *others* who also feel this same aloneness, and together in full *unconscious* cooperation we all further exacerbate this illusion of separateness.

The only way out of this mess is to turn inward: to get to "know thyself" as commanded by the oracle of Delphi. As we slowly discover what we are not, we eventually uncover true or Core Self—the unchanging essence which is attached to nothing (nothing) and from which everything flows.

The quickest (or shortest) way to Self-Knowledge is direct self-inquiry. By constantly going within and asking, *Who's angry? Who wants to know? Who is frustrated? Who is sad? Who loves? Who is laughing?*, we discover that nothing is there. After you go through all the standard labels of who you think is there, that you always call yourself, you discover a silent presence which is ultimately the only thing we ever need to be in relationship with. When we are in contact with this essence, we are then in touch with it in all others, no matter how they may be acting outwardly at the time. When you can live from this quiet presence, you no longer take your (or any one else's) persona seriously, and you seldom ever get hooked on needing to be right, on blame, guilt, fear, or the innumerable thought forms which habitually keep us hooked on the wheel of life.

Ultimately, to experience an abundance of love in our relationships, we need to see "others" as the true mirrors of Self that they really are. Each has the innate freedom and access to love and abundance as the next.

To see others in this light we first have to see ourselves. Our very awareness of true Self as the *source* of loving relationship is what enables us to *be* in loving relationship. To gain this awareness it is essential that we learn to feel our needs fully. By turning to our heartfelt need, true Self reveals itself.

## Abundance of Wealth

✓True wealth is a state of mind. In just the same way that we project our beliefs about another's behavior and then attract that same behavior in the other, the wealth or seeming lack of it we experience, is also a reflection of our projected beliefs. The ability to magnetize abundance is simply a matter of switching from a consciousness of negativity and lack to a new focus and concentration on wealth.

Most people are entirely unaware of how negative they really are when it comes to the issue of wealth and abundance. There are so many negative programs literally engulfing your poor mind all the time about the deleterious effect of money that it is not difficult to understand why the vast majority of people find themselves in lack. Because of all the negative beliefs about money, lack becomes the predominant feeling. As feelings are the greatest motivating factors in life, a feeling of lack will simply attract *more* of that same lack. In the *Core Abundance* seminar that I teach, we spend a lot of time in the first session uncovering all of the negative beliefs each individual carries about wealth. Unearthing your negative beliefs and exposing them to the light of truth, is an essential step in letting go and allowing abundance to finally flow through.

In the first 21 day process in this book, five minutes are spent each day just focusing on your resistance to the various issues of abundance in your life. As you feel your resistance and at the same time consider the beliefs which support this same resistance, you then create the space for desires to be fulfilled. The second five minutes are then spent putting all of your concentration on your heartfelt desires.

Heartfelt desires are the desires we feel at a gut level. They are the ones that always stay with us until they are addressed. Here, we differentiate clearly between fantasy or illusory desires which are impressed on us from the outside (and do not meet our deepest needs), and *heartfelt desires* which are Core Self speaking through the individual. True or Core Self which we all have in common, urges you to become more truly who you are; actually helps you fulfill your role in this life, by channeling to you the desires you need to motivate further growth. True or Core Self, however, is totally neutral as to whether our desires are actually fulfilled or not, thus it is entirely up to the individual to put his or her energy behind these desires and take action to see them through.

In actual fact true Self is the essence of each person individualized. Each "individual" true or Core Self magnetizes or creates the desires which will best produce in outward form the lessons the individual needs to learn, in order to move on and raise his or her Life Force Energy.

By following our desires, or as Joseph Campbell states, by following our bliss, we accomplish what we were put on this earth to do. When we follow our bliss, we put ourselves on a kind of track which has been there all the while, waiting for us, and then the life that we ought to have been living, becomes the one that we are living. Through the positive feelings which are evoked when we engage ourselves in activities that fulfill us, we expand our energy field. As the energy field is raised, our field of influence increases, and with that our abundance. We then begin to meet people who are in our field of bliss, and they open many doors for us.

To become abundant we simply have to feel abundant. We have to penetrate through all of our negative conditioning and get in touch with the unlimited Source that we are. We

54

simply have to convince the mind that we are abundant and we begin to attract that very same abundance.

Initially this may seem difficult as there seems to be so much "proof" in the world that "life is difficult", that "you have to work hard for your money" etc. How can I become abundant by simply changing my mind, when all around me "reality" tells me otherwise?

The truth is, that at present, most of humanity is still hypnotized by the mass consciousness (the collective unconscious described by Carl Jung) ideas of lack. Although it is so evident when you look at nature that there is incredible abundance, the united ego of mankind in mass hysteria about lack, rushes to destroy the planet in order to get its piece of the pie before it all "runs out".

This fear of lack is exactly what is killing us and destroying the environment. The root of greed is the fear that there is not enough to go around. I saw this amply illustrated in my own neighborhood in Washington state recently, when people started chopping down trees like crazy, as they feared new protective laws about to take effect, which would stop them from farming lumber as they pleased. We are at a point in the earth's history when we collectively need to take a major leap in faith, in the abundance which is already there just waiting for us to cultivate.

*When I was young*
*I knew Life to be a tree*
*and in the shade of its many branches*
*I enjoyed its fruit*
*Now*
*that I remember*
*the gate swings suddenly open*

Narayan

The belief that poverty is unavoidable, is reinforced by the unconscious people at the top of the social structure when they finance the further perpetration of this belief in lack through the mass media. In addition, the faithful of every religion are encouraged to donate to the poor. We are taught to have sympathy for the poor, while missing the whole point that to have sympathy or feel sorry for someone is one of the sickest ego trips on earth. When we feel sorry for someone, we are putting ourselves above that person. We buy into the belief that they are not as smart or intelligent or as fortunate as we are. Unfortunately, most of the poor buy into this belief as well, and the cycle continues. It is one thing to *empathize* with a fellow human being's unfortunate situation; to really *feel* and share what is needed to help them get back on their own feet. It is quite another to indulge in the insidious one-upmanship of sympathy.

The best thing we can do to help alleviate this situation and create a new reality for ourselves is simply to step outside of the beliefs of mainstream society. What is needed is a commitment to put some intense focus on the reality of abundance, and engage our minds in a whole new way of thinking. We need to disengage from all the negative emotions we have about money and wealth, and begin to focus instead on all the potential in ourselves and others. The two 21-day abundance plans in this book when completed with strong focus and intention will ensure this change of consciousness occurs.

As mass consciousness is very strong and the negative thoughts of others around us penetrate the subconscious mind constantly, it is important to periodically reinforce our new awareness with the ideas of abundance. If you find that certain areas in the plan evoke greater resistance for you, it might be wise to reinforce your new understanding periodically with a review of the resisted issues. Also recommended is reading other books on abundance to further reinforce your new awareness. One of my favorite books on this subject is Stuart Wilde's

*The Trick to Money Is Having Some.* He hilariously describes how we get caught up in "tick-tock" (the humdrum of everyday life), and forget that money-making is *not* a serious business, that it is actually a game that you play. He helps you to see that although it may seem that it is a game you play with forces outside of yourself—the economies of the market place, so to speak—what you actually discover is that it is a game you play with yourself. Wayne Dyer's *Real Magic* is also very helpful, along with John Randolf Price's *Abundance Book*, which helped me change my own ideas about lack seven years ago, and inspired me to create my own abundance plan.

Most important for creating wealth and developing a prosperity consciousness in your life is the decision to trust in the universe. As we have seen, this is not an easy task with most of society simultaneously engaged in a major deficit of trust, often operating on the totally opposite polarity of worry.

One of the five Reiki principles, "just for today, I will not worry", is a good guideline to follow in order to keep this focus on trust. Worry only happens when we forget that there is a Divine or Universal purpose in everything. When we maintain contact with true or Core Self, and from a space of silent mind live each day to the best of our ability, we are then aware that we have done everything in our power that we possibly can, and the rest is up to Universal Life Force. Worry is a thought pattern which results in a feeling of separateness from true or Core Self, from the *I AM* consciousness of Universal Wholeness. It comes from being identified with the illusory "I" and its elaborate support system of judgments and beliefs. To eradicate this identification, direct self-enquiry is recommended. For further insights into this process *Wake Up And Roar I* and *II* by H.W.L. Poonja is an excellent introduction.

To worry about the past is futile. It helps to remember that each person (including ourselves) does the best that he or she can, in each of life's situations, in accordance with the knowledge or wisdom that he or she has at any given moment. We are all products of our conditioning and most often react according to our past experience. If you regret a past action, it helps to realize that you reacted according to your resources at that time; then, be thankful for the lesson and move on. It is essential to also realize that all injustices done to you in the past were done by others as a result of their conditioning. It is wise to wish them well (to forgive them and ourselves), and have faith that they, too, have learned from their actions.

To worry needlessly about the future is also futile. There is a saying I live by: "Expect the best in life and when you receive something you didn't expect, know and trust that it is the best for you in your present situation." Even if at the time something happens, it seems very negative, it is only a lesson. Somehow I helped magnetize the situation, even if on a subconscious level, to learn. I consciously choose to feel gratitude that it has come to pass, and that I am now free. Then I move on.

What works for me, is to surrender to true Self and try not to interfere with the Universal timing in life. I know that in my perfect flow, when I am following my heartfelt desire, there is a certain synchronicity of events. As long as I have completed my role in the scheme of things, all else is taken care of. Worrying results from illogical and irrational patterns of thought; it is totally fear based. It creates more limitations, and in turn, a further separation in consciousness.

When I first became a Reiki master, and started teaching, it took a major leap of faith in the Universe to do so. I had just finished graduate school, and had received strong inner guidance that it was my role to share all of the things I had learned on the road. I had accumulated quite a storehouse of knowledge, and I was instructed to go out into the world and "empty my cup". I was informed it wasn't so important what I taught, as how I taught it. The essential point was that whatever I taught should come straight from the heart. People would not remember so much what I said, as they would the heart energy that was behind it.

As I set out in my car across the U.S. with a few contacts to get me started, I had no idea how things would turn out. Sometimes, courses I had expected would be full, simply fell apart. At other times, as the result of "chance" meetings, other courses happened quite by "accident", enabling me to fulfill all my financial obligations. Over the years I really learned to relax no matter how things turned out. It became very clear that certain people were meant to come together in a particular group and at a certain time. Sometimes it was a small group and sometimes a large group, but whichever way it turned out was totally appropriate in the moment. I began to notice how each group would "draw" certain teachings through me. As they asked questions, I also learned from the answers that were evoked.

The more I surrendered to the process of teaching and let go of my preconceived notions of how things "should" go, the richer my life became. Slowly but surely I lost my worries about money. Somehow the bills always got paid, and I even had extra to splurge when I needed to treat myself. Soon, I decided to return to Europe where I had spent many of my childhood years, and there my contacts also grew. Finally, I realized I was playing the role I had unknowingly been groomed for, to teach and network in a variety of cultures.

By doing what I really enjoy, it seems I also have been able to bring a lot of joy to others. In my travels around the world, I have found that this is the key to wealth: to do what you enjoy, and to do it well. If you find fulfillment in your work, others will feel your positive energy and want to share in it no matter what it is you do.

This works on an individual scale, as well as in a large company. I recall my two years as a spa director on a cruise ship. The first two captains were lovely, cultured men. Both were sensitive, yet very self confident; they could delegate easily and trusted the crew and staff to do their jobs with little interference. While they were on board, the crew and staff were very happy, and the passengers, feeling our comradship, encouraged their friends to also cruise with us. After these two wonderful captains, we were then forced to deal with two real duds. The third captain was a total alcoholic and had to quit due to cirrhosis of the liver. The fourth was hoodwinked by a nasty, controlling head housekeeper into "laying down the law" by creating all kinds of unfair and needless regulations. The morale of the staff and crew deteriorated rapidly, and our business with it. It was like a Loveboat version of "Mutiny on the Bounty". I quit as soon as I got one Alaska trip out of it, as did several other key people.

My experience on board taught me several things, the most important being that what people need most, is approval. The crew needed to feel the approval of the captain. In turn, the passengers needed to feel that they were appreciated by the crew. Everything flowed well, as long as approval filtered down from the top. As soon as the crew became disgruntled, they could no longer patiently handle the occasional belligerent passenger, and soon all passengers began to look like "cattle" to be processed for the week. One insecurity just initiated another. What I learned from this experience, is that what you have to do to be successful in any business, is find out what people need, and then give it to them.

What people need in addition to approval, is a feeling of security. If you can help them feel secure, even if on a temporary basis by giving them healing words, by being willing to serve them, you will be a great success in your business. By creating a relaxed, positive environment, people will flock to you. Then all you have to do is bill them. This may be a harder task for women at first, as we are so brainwashed to giving service for free. With practice though, it becomes easier. When you realize your own worth, people feel your self confidence, and they react to it accordingly.

To really feel your own worth, at some point you have to give up your own need for approval from others. If you are still trying internally to please Mom and Dad or your spouse or family, you are not free. It will be difficult to genuinely serve others, as you will still be stuck in your own neediness. Instead of being able to serve your client or customer, on an unconscious level, you will be seeking approval from them, and they will easily pick up on it. This applies as well to all the other relationships in your life. Even those closest to you will unconsciously play on your need for approval, in order to get what they want from you in the moment.

In the long run, people actually prefer to be with others who don't need their approval, as a secure person is much more giving in a real genuine sense. A secure person is one who is very much in tune with true Self, the very core of Being, and therefore connects with others on the same level.

You can feel when someone doesn't have an agenda for you, and accepts you just as you are, simply because you are you (another aspect of true Self). You automatically want to give back to such a person, as they evoke the natural generosity you were born with, but may have temporarily forgotten. It is clear to see why such a person would attract wealth easily. They are totally open to whatever is there in the moment. For abundance of wealth, openness is a necessity. To receive this wealth, you only have to open to it in each moment. It is simply a choice of beingness: To be or not to be, that is the question.

# Abundance of Experience

When you accept wealth as the simple flow of Universal Life Force Energy that it is, you open yourself up to a myriad of possibilities. In all of the various spiritual traditions, it is easy to see that most enlightened masters dissolved their final attachment to the I (which had kept them separate from what they longed for for so long) only after having sampled a wide variety of life's experiences. To be ready to dissolve your many attachments and let go of your desires, it may first be necessary to fulfill them. Buddha was a prince who had experienced many of life's pleasures. Mohammed, although the prophet of the one and only God, throughout his life remained a man of the world. Jesus, who was also very worldly, traveled widely and is thought to have studied in the Egyptian mystery schools and with a variety of Eastern masters. St. Francis of Assisi is another example of an experienced wealthy nobleman, who later gave up his attachment to money, to live simply. My own teacher, H.W.L. Poonja was quite a man of the world with many varied experiences behind him before he recognized his unity with true Self.

The important point to note here, is that money itself was not a hindrance on the path, for the most part they simply transcended the need for it. They were neither for nor against it. In his teachings, Jesus would admonish the rich not to chase after or covet money, and he would encourage the poor that wealth and abundance were everywhere available. The message inherent in all the teachings is quite practical; simply to find balance, to neither be for nor against money.

To be able to reach the point where you can finally let go of your attachments, so that they fall away of their own accord, you may have to complete certain life experiences. Sometimes to complete these experiences you may need money. The secret is to focus your intention on the experience you want to carry out (rather than the money per se) and the funds or necessary resources will certainly manifest. It is important to then take action to accomplish what your heart desires.

Once you have established a consciousness of abundance, it is important to keep your mind focused on what it is you want to complete in your life. It is essential to stay in tune with your heartfelt desires and follow through with the steps you need to take, to make them come true. The key thing is to make a decision as to what you want, and then go for it. You need to also then put your energy behind it one hundred percent.

The vast majority of people unfortunately suffer from what I call "decidophobia". They spend their entire lives being swayed by one idea after another. "Oh, wouldn't it be nice, if I could do this?" "Oh, wouldn't it be nice, if I could do that" So many people waste their entire lives caught up in illusory hopes and wishful thoughts; an unending list of "what ifs", constantly distracting them from their true potential until it is really too late, as death is at their very doorstep.

Hope is one of the other useless states of mind we are programmed with, which often keeps us from our true potential and feeds decidophobia. When we invest our energy in hoping for a better future, we continue to mentally place our good always one step ahead of us—in the future. We end up always being one step away from what we want. What we need to realize is that there is actually no past or future, there is only one eternal present. If you aren't having a good time now, chances are you won't be either a few moments down the line. Abundance only happens now. We have to keep recreating it in the *now*.

By focusing on what we want in our lives, and putting our energies and actions wholeheartedly behind our choices, we release our need for the illusion of hope, as we are then totally engaged in the joyful process of the moment.

As we release the need for hope, because we begin to see how easy it is to manifest whatever we want in physical reality, we then enable ourselves to step one step closer to freedom from desire or the state of "want".

A really good example of ease of manifestation, is a recent discussion I had with one of my students in Australia who participated in the *Core Empowerment Training* that I also teach around the world. At the very beginning of *C.E.T.*, we stress the importance of getting in touch with what it is you want in life, then choosing it, and formulating a course of action to ensure results. Our ultimate "goal" though, is to eventually transcend even the need for goals. However, it is first necessary to experience your ability to manifest what it is you need in your life. To go beyond the average human being's fear for survival, it is essential to experience a consistent natural flow of abundance at some point of your life.

The woman I spoke with had kept a picture book of her goals for five years. Very systematically, she had daily meditated on her goals and, using pictures from magazines and other sources, she visualized consistently along with a support group of like minded others, the goals she wished to manifest in reality. Over a five year period, she had methodically created the house of her dreams on the beach, sold her old business, started a new career and completed a variety of other goals on her list. Because of her experience, of being able to easily manifest her intentions into physical reality, she could now let go and really trust the universe to present to her in each moment, what was most appropriate for her. No longer attached to her desires or ego, she was able to let go and allow Universal Life Force Energy to work though her.

Through her experiences and willingness to receive the abundance of the universe, she gained greater trust in true Self. It may be important to experience this flow in order to become well rounded. We may need to go after our heartfelt desires and pursue them until they naturally fall away. With enough experiences and adventure under your belt, the adrenaline rush you received initially begins to loose its appeal. As you fulfill each desire, eventually it also becomes clear how one desire, when complete, leads to another.

As you begin to perceive this constant flow of desires through the mind, it becomes easier to let go and allow them to flow through you without any hooks. To reach the state where you are neither for nor against desire, you may need a broad range of experience, so that even "experience" is no longer a hook. We then learn to just *be* with each moment, no longer attached to any certain outcome. When we are no longer attached to any particular outcome, we are free to be in total awe of the moment, much like a little child of two or three, who is captured by whatever he is involved with in each instant. There is no longer any past or future, simply total wonderment in the moment.

To be in total abundance, we have to cultivate the ability to be in the moment. Opening ourselves to a great variety of experiences may be a powerful step toward that end. Experiencing life's many situations with a sense of wonderment will certainly bring us further into that moment and into our true abundance.

Chapter 4

# The 42-Day Program
# To Core Abundance

After having formulated the exact steps of the 21-day plans which are to be completed one after the other in an uninterrupted 42 day time span, I was excited to see how well the numbers work together numerologically. The two 21-day plans correspond interestingly to the 21 day cleansing process which occurs after receiving the Reiki attunements, and also to the 21 days Dr. Usui spent on the mountain in his own personal quest. Each 21-day plan has three seven day cycles, and according to mystic law, to state anything from Source three times makes it truth (the law of three).

The number 42 itself is considered an auspicious sign in several traditions. According to Linda Goodman's interpretation of the numerology of the Kabbalah, 42 is one of the luckiest numbers there are. It is the number of Love, Money, and Creativity, and symbolizes karmic reward. 42 signifies that you can now finally harvest the seeds that you have sown. Its greatest attribute is the many blessings it bestows to help you manifest what you have been preparing for during previous incarnations. The important point when working with the number 42 (and in life in general), is that you do not gloat over what now comes to you so easily. Instead it is recommended that you take the opportunity to merge even further with the grace of Universal Life Force Energy.

In the Chinese *I Ching* or *Book of Changes*, 42 symbolizes *Increase*. In the various commentaries on hexagram 42, it is said that it would be "advantageous to have a goal, and to cross the great river". As the image suggests, you transcend

67

ordinary limitations and learn to trust in the waters of life. "Crossing the great river" points toward a process of initiation into a greater life: You leave the old shore behind and establish yourself on totally new ground. It is also mentioned that all obstacles have now been cleared away, that Heaven gives abundantly and that Earth bears rich harvest. There is a time for abundance, and this time is the eternal *NOW.*

Another author, Stephan Endres, in his groundbreaking introduction to numbers in different mythologies, links 42 to the number 40 which plays an important role in several spiritual traditions such as in Christianity and Sufism, the esoteric school of Islam. He mentions that similar to Jesus' 40 days in the desert, the traditional Sufi retreat also takes place over 40 days. These and many other examples point to the fact that 40 (or 42) days have long been considered a timespan ideal for raising your Life Force Energy and making major changes in consciousness.

## Dissolving Lack

In order to experience abundance, it is necessary to first get in touch with what is keeping you in lack. The first 21 days of your 42 day program are designed to help dissolve the feeling of not having enough in different areas of your life. The intention of the first half of the program is to help you overcome any ambivalence and get in touch with the polarity consciousness which has held it in place. Each day, is completed with the attitude of gratitude to help alleviate this same polarized thinking.

Desire and resistance are the basic forces fueling our ordinary experience. We desire what we feel will bring us pleasure or happiness, and we resist whatever we perceive to be its opposite.

Each day resistance is addressed first, as resistance is what keeps us from being open to a natural flow of abundance. The other polarity, desire, is then addressed. As long as there is desire, resistance remains. As long as there is resistance, there is also desire. One is the shadow side of the other, and they both infer lack. Resistance does so explicitly by shunning the creative forces that express abundance. Desire implicitly infers lack, because by desiring you imply to yourself that you don't already have—that you are lacking. Therefore, resistance and desire for a certain quality have to be dissipated before this quality can manifest in its authentic form.

In the course of the first 21-day plan you will experience your resistance and desire for seven basic qualities. They are related to the seven subtle energy centers and as such are blueprints for the patterns that dominate your life. By dissolving the blueprints which hold you in a state of lack, you open yourself enough to be able to gratefully acknowledge the *transforming presence* of the very same qualities you used to desire and resist.

## Complete Abundance

The second 21 days provide an unprecedented opportunity for you to directly access Unity. Instead of remaining oblivious and in lack, you merge with the vast and abundant ocean of consciousness by concentrating on seven powerful statements of Reality.

These statements are tailored to direct you toward the possibility of experiencing a silence beyond mind. By going deeply into the simple yet basic question, "Who am I?", we gain access to the silent Divine Presence which has been there all along—true or Core Self which is the no-thing and provider of everything that I AM. When we gain access to this inner silence, questions of abundance are no longer pertinent, as we come to understand that *we are that abundance*. The various thoughts which have disturbed our peace, although still there, no longer hook our attention. If we do get temporarily distracted, we can now easily return to source.

## A Time to Focus

Ninty nine percent of the time your consciousness is not in focus. Instead, thousands of thoughts are passing through your mind at random. These are not original thoughts, as they arise from past memories and future plans. As long as you are attached to these thoughts, they will constantly grab your attention and drain your power. Always reinforcing your past conditioning even further, they are bound to keep you in the very state of lack that has been programmed into you.

If you want to break free of the forces that bind you and rob you of your precious energy, you will need to surrender to the natural flow of relaxed concentration which happens within Universal Life Force Energy. To facilitate this flow, you can also support the first 21-day plan by giving Reiki to the appropriate energy center each day as you concentrate on your feelings. During the second 21-day plan it is recommended that you give Reiki to your heart, or simply follow your intention in the moment. It is not absolutely essential to have received the Reiki attunements in order to do the program. Reiki is simply a powerful tool to help accentuate the process.

The first 21-day plan addresses issues similar to First Degree Reiki. Like First Degree Reiki, which dissolves imbalances on a more physical and emotional level, the first 21-day plan clears away the coarser obstacles to abundance. It helps you neutralize the resistance and desire which otherwise keep your consciousness within the walled enclosure of duality. As long as your mind is hooked between the polarity of resistance and desire, you are bound to be jostled back and forth between the two, never fulfilling your desires because of your conscious or unconscious resistance, yet desiring all the same what you feel you cannot have. By feeling them and putting all of our awareness on these two we help to dissipate them. By feeling them with love and enthusiasm (even and especially the negative aspects), we help break through the various levels of emotional resistance which keeps these two in place. You also address the key assumptions that have kept you on this merry go round of resistance and desire, until their hold on you is relaxed and finally broken. Five minutes are then spent in focused gratitude to further help remind you of the abundance which has always been a part of your life.

The second 21-day plan helps to deepen your experience of abundance and puts you in touch with even finer energies. Here you focus on the reality of non-duality. In a sense, you are projecting yourself into the realm where there is no more separation. The intention of the second 21-day plan to *Core Abundance* can be likened to Second Degree Reiki which by transcending the limits of time and space promotes a greater sense of Unity. Further practice will ground you in this new reality of the paradox of there being no goals and yet there being tremendous (and tremendously liberating) results. Whatever you do, it actually comes to you—by virtue of the fact that you already are *THAT*. To the ordinary mind this may appear to be magic; in reality it is only the simple application of the laws of non-duality.

## How to Approach the 42-Day Program

You need to follow just a few basic guidelines and take into account the four factors of **desire**, **commitment**, **consistancy**, and **detachment** in order to make your effort with the two 21-day plans to *Core Abundance* truly successful.

The first important factor is **desire**. Desire is a tightrope issue. On the one hand, you want to transcend or simply drop the kind of desires which are not really yours, but implants of your conditioning. On the other hand you need a strong desire to mobilize the forces that can help you break free from the conditioning that has perpetuated your experience of lack. In order to open to the abundant presence of Life Force Energy that is available to you by virtue of the role you have come to play, you need a strong desire to live in such abundance. Also, you are already "supplied with" a number of very specific desires, which will guide you toward the lessons you came here to learn, but most importantly what you need to cultivate, is the desire to be free. Without this strong desire, liberation is next to impossible. Therefore, become aware of your desire. Feel your desire for living in the abundance of Self, and use it well.

The second factor is **commitment**. A half-hearted approach at any stage of the program will sabotage your results. An attitude such as: "Oh well, maybe I should try this, too. I'll see, if it works for me, and if it doesn't, nothing is lost." will get you nowhere fast. This attitude will not help you attain anything in life, or wake you up to the hard fact of your present existence and to what is controlling your every move: your years of conditioning. To energize this program and make it really powerful for yourself, you have to make a clear decision and then follow through.

In one respect, these plans are like all the others you want to realize in life. To make a start you have to give your word. You have to declare: "This is done!" As soon as you make that statement to yourself or to others, it is important to live up to your word. If you don't, you undermine your own ability to achieve your goals. You then dissipate your power. Eventually you end up invalidating yourself to the point where you don't believe your own words, and who else will believe you, if you can't even believe yourself?

The third factor is **consistency**. Once you are commited, in order to to experience results, you will need to complete both 21-day plans without missing one step. If for any reason you forget your abundance practice at any point, it is important to start the entire 42-day program once more from the beginning. It is crucial that you finish both plans in one continous flow; that you work on them for 42 consecutive days! If you miss even one day, results can no longer be guaranteed, as the momentum necessary to break the force of habit and conditioning will be interrupted. The two plans are a step-by-step program. If you leave out one step, you will tumble down the whole length of the ladder.

**Detachment**, the fourth factor, is also very important. It infers, that you are not attached as to how abundance will manifest in your life. Fully realizing that you are not trying to change anything; you put your trust in the Universe, and allow Universal Life Force Energy to provide in an infinite number of ways. There is a certain paradox involved in detachment. On the one hand, you can be very specific in formulating your goals. You know exactly what you want: what kind of relationship, what kind of career, what amount of income, what kind of house and where and so on. On the other hand, you do *not* insist that everything be delivered according to plan. You open yourself to receiving what could turn out to be even better than what are able to conceive of now. The point of being clear about your desires is that you automatically put out the right kind of energy in order to attract your highest good, and through your detachment there is a certain trust which insures you receive that which you have intended. You are also naturally open to receiving. Abundance is continually attracted to those who are clear about what they want (and on a certain level already have), and are not attached to the various ways it manifests.

With **desire, commitment, consistancy** and **detachment** clearly at your fingertips, you are now ready to immerse yourself in the two 21-day plans that will totally change the way you perceive your life.

## *Beginning the 21-Day Plan to Dissolving Lack*

In order to live in abundance, you need to get in touch with the beliefs that separate you from this aspect of yourself. You have to become very clear about what has prevented you from continually abiding in this fundamental state of Being which is your actual birthright. Questions such as, "Why do I often do the exact opposite of what I originally set out to do?" "How does my desire for one particular thing very often ensure that I remain in lack?" "Why do I so often sabotage my own best intentions and harm my own best interests?" "How can I dissolve lack?" The answer to all these questions is very simple: You don't *feel* abundant, and you have to *feel* abundant, in order to *be* abundant.In order to feel abundant, we have to first deal with our unconscious resistance to abundance, and we have to also address the desires that feed this resistance and keep it alive.

The root of our problem is that we are lost in polarity consciousness, and true abundance transcends polarity. It is a state of beingness *beyond* polarity. True abundance is all encompassing and can grant the satisfaction that particular entities (such as persons and events) cannot grant. The human mind of everyday conditioned existence, on the other hand, is totally enmeshed in polarities, which is exactly why the mind cannot create abundance. To access the state of abundance we have to move beyond mind. A major step in this direction, is to get out of your head (which only keeps you in a state of trying to figure things out), and focus on your heart which contains the feelings that put you in touch with everything you need to know.

The human mind (our judgments, beliefs and survival games) sets up the very walls that keep us from enjoying true abundance. It is the very breeding ground for lack. There is no need to despair, however, because what is there, is there for a reason. At one point in our development, as in childhood or adolescence, we needed those same judgments and beliefs in order to survive, although they are what also now keeps our sense of lack in place. Whenever our inner call becomes strong enough, however, we have the ability to clear away all the obstacles to abundance. We are not condemned to restriction forever, as it is only a temporary learning tool. What we can do, is cultivate the attitude of gratitude with full-bodied enthusiasm.

Enthusiasm is an essential ingredient to dissolving our attachment to our judgments, beliefs, emotions and experience. We all share the natural tendency to avoid painful memories or emotions that upset us. These thoughtforms crystallize in the body, but can actually be dissolved when we are in a true state of full-bodied enthusiasm or ecstasy. In exciting research at Stanford University scientists discovered that when we are enthusiastic the brain puts out certain chemicals which dissolve melanin protein complex (which is effected by the stimulus response mechanism). Melanin is very likely what crystallizes and blocks our cells every time we make a judgment, which then prevents the possibility for an all pervasive knowledge from flowing through. Perhaps, the only difference between an ordinary being and an enlightened being, is that the cells of an enlightened being are fully open for all knowledge and abundance to flow through, contrary to ours which are blocked by our judgments and beliefs.

During the next 21 days it is very important to imbue the entire process with enthusiasm. You need to feel all of your feelings *fully* with enthusiasm, regardless as to whether they are positive or *negative*. Each day you will experience a simple three stage process of addressing all basic forms of (1) your resistance to abundance, (2) the desire you feel—and (3) cultivating gratitude for the abundance in seven major areas of your life which are interrelated with the issues of the seven main chakras.

When working with these seven steps it is important to practice them according to instruction. You begin with step one on the first day for 15 minutes, step two on the second day for 15 minutes and so on until on the seventh day, the first cycle is complete. On day eight, you start the second cycle of seven steps, and on day fifteen the third until all twenty one days are complete. On the twenty-second day, you immediately begin the second *21-Day Plan To Complete Abundance*.

During the entire 42 day period it is essential that you keep a journal and record your feelings and reactions, immediately after each session, taking special note of particularly resistant areas. Later after the 42 day program is complete, it is wise to occasionally repeat the steps where you felt the most resistance. This will keep you from falling prey to the mass consciousness of limited beliefs in these areas.

To ensure that you do not miss a session, it is recommended that you choose a specific time of day that you know will work best for you in the long run. The time after awakening each morning is ideal, as it sets the whole tone of your day with the attitude of gratitude and a feeling of full-bodied enthusiasm.

# A 21-Day Plan
# To
# Dissolving Lack

# Step 1
## (Day 1, 8, and 15)

*Experience the thoughts*
*and resulting emotions*
*that block the flow of abundance*
*in the first or root chakra*

Sit in a comfortable position, your spine erect, yet relaxed, your ears over your shoulders and your shoulders over your hips,
> *for 5 minutes*
> *feel all of your resistance to abundance;*

Experience fully with complete *enthusiasm* all of your negative thoughts about abundance, such as: "Life is difficult." "You have to work hard for your money." Or, "Money is the root of all evil."

Recall incidents when your beliefs were proved "true". Now, experience the resulting emotions throughout the entire body and expand until they dissipate.

Now,
> *for 5 minutes,*
> *feel your desire for all the things*
> *you want in your life.*

Experience them fully, with complete *enthusiasm*. Recall all of your desires, all of your wishes, and all of your goals for the future. Now, experience the resulting emotions throughout the entire body and expand until they dissipate.

Finally,
> *for 5 minutes*
> *feel gratitude*
> *for the richness in your life now.*

Explore your gratitude for all the abundance that has already manifested in your life; the things you own, your personal experiences and your friends and loved ones. Experience it fully, with complete *enthusiasm.*

After you are complete, carry this attitude of gratitude into your daily activities. Let the attitude of gratitude touch whatever you have to do or accomplish during this truly wonderful and glorious day.

## Commentary

All abundance issues are particularly connected to blockages in the root chakra, because this is the energy center where spirit and matter are linked. The root chakra deals with physical manifestation. Located at the lower end of the spine, the root chakra's primary function is to manifest the physical expression of Universal Life Force Energy. As the Sanskrit word (*muladhara*) for this energy center suggests, it is the "base of everything" (*mula*=root; *adhara*=support). When the base malfunctions, everything malfunctions, as abundance cannot unfold without support.

We can turn this situation around by simply allowing our true thoughts and emotions to surface by directing all of our attention on them. By acknowledging what we feel, we no longer deny the tremendous resistance we have against abundance. Through our acknowledgment of these same feelings our resistance dissipates, and we are freed from the tendency to struggle.

By feeling our desires fully, we finally come to accept them and neutralize the hooks they have on consciousness. We can now encompass the heartfelt desires, which flow through us in order to gently guide us toward the lessons we came here to learn, while at the same time being aware of the danger that if we are not careful, we can begin to identify with them. On the one hand, they are as necessary for our development as the air we breathe, on the other, if we become *attached* to our desires, they undoubtedly lead us into suffering.

Finally we drop these polarities by dissolving both resistance and desire in the attitude of gratitude for the abundance which is already ours. The attitude of gratitude dissolves all sense of fear or need. As such it perfectly expresses natural abundance.

By energetically feeling both our resistance to abundance and our desire for abundance, we prepare the ground for abundance to manifest of its own accord. We open ourselves to the wisdom of not striving. We are now able to joyously accept all of what life offers, because we can now directly experience that life comes into being through the consciousness that we are.

# Step 2
## (Day 2, 9, and 16)

*Experience the thoughts*
*and resulting emotions*
*that block the flow of abundance*
*in the second or navel chakra*

Sit in a comfortable position, your spine erect, yet relaxed, your ears over your shoulders and your shoulders over your hips,
  *for 5 minutes*
    *feel all of your resistance to sex,*
    *and to expressing your feelings.*
Experience fully, with complete *enthusiasm* how rare it is to experience conscious connected sex. Also explore any fears you have about your feelings, or any difficulties expressing feelings.

Recall certain events which evoke these feelings for you clearly and intensify them. Now, experience the resulting emotions throughout the entire body and expand until they dissipate.

Now,

>for 5 minutes,
>feel your desire for sex,
>feeling, and expression of feeling.

Experience this desire fully, with complete *enthusiasm*. Note how often your desire for sex pervades your everyday life. Also examine some specific incidents where you had a strong desire to communicate your feelings, but felt inhibited. Experience what you felt throughout the body until it dissipates.

Finally,

>for 5 minutes
>feel gratitude for all the sexual experiences
>you have had in your life,
>including the ones you would label "negative".

Also experience the joy of heartfelt intimacy when you were able to express yourself deeply to another. Feel your gratitude for all your past sexual experiences; for the feelings you have had, and the way you were able to express them.

After you are complete, carry this attitude of gratitude into your feelings and expression of feelings. Let the attitude of gratitude touch you whenever you feel or express your feelings throughout the day.

# Commentary

All sexual issues, and issues dealing with feeling and the expression of feelings are in one way or another related to blockages in this energy center, because it is here that the water element of feeling is meant to unfold. Thus, the navel (or belly) chakra controls feeling, particulary sexual feelings and feelings in relationships. When feelings are blocked, we lose our natural flow of creativity.

Life began in water. When the waters of life are not in balance and harmony, life itself becomes threatened, and natural abundance cannot find appropriate ways to assert itself. The water element also symbolizes purification. Thus sex, when as truthful and innocent as unconditional love, and feelings when sincere, both have a purifying effect and contribute to living in abundance. As authentic expressions of Life Force Energy, they wash away hardened emotionality and other forces of stagnation.

For true feelings to happen and be expressed in our lives, we have to learn to be still and listen. We have to learn to distinguish between the true ease of underlying feelings, and the demanding, urgent neediness of emotion, caused by thoughts or belief in lack. The neediness of emotion creates huge walls of resistance against sexual and other feelings we desire to have.

However, when honestly and deeply feeling our resistance against sex and true feelings, our very focus acts to dissolve the resistance.

Resistance and desire for sex and true feelings, eventually create imbalances in the endocrine system, which in turn psychologically manifest in the form of seemingly endless difficulties in all of our relationships. All of these difficulties mirror emotional patterns in ourselves that until now have remained unconscious or unacknowledged.

84

Experiencing them fully as resistance and then desire will finally liberate us from their grip, and also open us to the possibility of true relationship.

# Step 3

(Day 3, 10, and 17)

*Experience the thoughts
and resulting emotions
that block the flow of abundance
in the third or solar plexus chakra*

Sit in a comfortable position, your spine erect, yet relaxed, your ears over your shoulders and your shoulders over your hips,

*for 5 minutes
feel all of your resistance to
your own power and wisdom.*

Experience fully, with complete *enthusiasm* any difficulties you have being with your own power and wisdom, and any fear you may have about asserting them. Consider also how often you use the phrase "I don't know.", or "I know."

Recall any resentment you have about others who have tried to control you, or incidents when you were controlling. Feel the emotions you felt during these experiences throughout the entire body and expand until they dissipate.

Now,
   *for 5 minutes,*
   *feel any desire you have*
   *to express your own power and wisdom.*

Experience this desire fully, with complete *enthusiasm,* feeling fully your desire to contact your own inner power and wisdom. Recall specific incidents when you were unsure about your abilities. Now, experience the resulting emotions throughout the entire body and expand until they dissipate.

Finally,
   *for 5 minutes*
   *contemplate all the experiences*
   *you have had in your life being and asserting*
   *your own power and wisdom.*

Feel deeply grateful for all your past experiences, for the power and wisdom you have had, and the way in which you were able to express them.

After you are complete, on a daily basis bring the attitude of gratitude into your expression of power and wisdom. Let the attitude of gratitude touch you whenever you feel or express your power and wisdom during the day.

# Commentary

All power and wisdom issues are particularly connected to blockages in this energy center, because it is in the solar plexus chakra where our "internal sun" or power center is meant to shine forth. The solar plexus chakra nourishes both etheric and physical bodies alike.

Here, Universal Life Force Energy starts to interact with the outer world. Thus, in this energy center the will to shape, form, and fashion needs to be appreciated. It needs to find many different ways to express itself. It is therefore plain to see that any blockages in this center also automatically block the flow of abundance in our lives.

To be abundant, we have to encompass the masculine quality of sheer determination. To enjoy fullness and completion in our lives, we also need the feminine quality of satisfying our deep and heartfelt desires by acceptance. Both of these are qualities of the solar plexus chakra. Together they help us accomplish transformation by acting wisely and with self-confidence.

The more our energy is allowed to flow naturally through the solar plexus chakra, the more we are able to actively engage in life with the power and wisdom that is uniquely ours. Also the more power and wisdom we are able to express, the less resistance we develop against our own, and the power and wisdom of others.

In order to break any apparent deadlock against our inner wisdom and power, we only have to have the courage to face our true feelings. We have to be willing to experience fully with *enthusiasm* our strong resistance against our own power and wisdom.

Resistance is easy to spot. It shows itself in the urge to control and manipulate, and in the almost despairing drive for recognition and material gain which results in the opposite of what it attempts to achieve. He who attempts to act by controlling everything ends up being totally controlled. As the Taoist sage Chuang Tzu states: "He who acts upon an (emotionally preset) agenda, makes himself available to the world and suffers lack. He who acts without being (emotionally) involved, has all the world available to him and enjoys abundance."

In part two, we also accept our desire for power and wisdom. This desire motivates us. It is the same desire that fuels evolution. There are unique occasions and important junctures in every life, when we really need to follow our heartfelt desire. Our desire does not have to be "spiritual" in order to be valid, because, *when heartfelt,* every desire eventually leads far beyond its own limitations.

In this way, your desire for power and wisdom, when heartfelt, turns into devotion. In true devotion no action or purification of action is necessary. As H.W.L. Poonja states: "In devotion you surrender to the Supreme. You do nothing but surrender to the Supreme, who will look after everything, as it does even now."

In surrender, an abundance of power and wisdom unfold, but there is no one there, who claims: "I did that." To be grateful for all instances of power and wisdom in your life is a first step to such abundance, although, ultimately, there are not successive steps leading to abundance. Abundance of power and wisdom is already here. You just have to plunge in and see.

# Step 4
### (Day 4, 11, and 18)

*Experience the thoughts*
*and resulting emotions*
*that block the flow of abundance*
*in the fourth or heart chakra.*

Sit in a comfortable position, your spine erect, yet relaxed, your ears over your shoulders and your shoulders over your hips,
> *for 5 minutes*
> *feel all your resistance to unconditional love,*
> *feel any feelings you have*
> *that you are unworthy of receiving love.*

Experience fully, with complete *enthusiasm* how difficult it is to feel unconditional love, and how much you are afraid to love unconditionally.

Recall incidents in relationship, where out of fear of vulnerability, you pushed others away. Feel all the emotions you felt throughout your entire body and expand until they dissipate.

Now,
*for 5 minutes,*
*feel your desire for approval*
*and for unconditional love.*

Experience this desire fully, with complete *enthusiasm*, feeling fully your need for approval and how much you want to experience true unconditional love.

Recall incidents when you have compromised yourself to gain approval. Feel the resulting emotions throughout your entire body and expand until they dissipate.

Finally,
*for 5 minutes*
*contemplate all the instances in your life,*
*when you encountered true and unconditional love.*

Feel deeply grateful for all your past experiences of unconditional love, those moments when love was given or received without a thought of "What's in it for me?".

After you are complete, carry this attitude of gratitude into the way you feel and express love. Let the attitude of gratitude touch you whenever you feel or express love during the day.

# Commentary

We are living at a time in the history of our planet, when incredible amounts of love energy are engulfing us, opening us to the unity of all creation. This love energy needs an open heart to be experienced without pain. When confronted with a closed heart, this incredible surplus of love energy, which is permeating the earth, finds expression in turmoil, conflict and illness. The many civil wars around the globe are a sign that our hearts have not yet opened enough to receive the abundance of love that now wants to enter the lives of our earth family. Illnesses of the heart and the immune system are yet another sign of the same healing crisis that we are undergoing collectively. All of these show our resistance to love, and the simplest way to dissolve such resistance is by acknowledging it.

Abundance does not exist without love. The same way the fourth chakra is central to all energy centers, love energy is the central energy of the universe. If you wish to experience an abundance of love, you first must be willing to feel all your resistance against love. Really go deep into all your feelings of unworthiness, your deep need for approval, and any ideas you have which negate love. Examine your fear of vulnerability, of how you might be hurt if you open your heart.

Experience how you are embarassed and confused when confronted with true love. Feel those feelings of unfamiliarity, of hinderance, of some sort of imminent danger. Feel how you reject love, and then how you are absolutely starved for love, because you don't dare open up to love.

If you open enough to feel your resistance and desire for love, this true and unconditional love will reveal itself to you. You will know love intimately. Love doesn't *happen* to you. You don't depend on outside sources to hand out rations of love, because, by feeling love, you recognize that you *are* the source of limitless love.

All issues of true love, of empathy with living things are

closely related to the opening of this energy center, because it is here where the more "physical" and "emotional" forces of the "lower" energy centers meet with the more "refined" forces of the "higher" energy centers.

Whenever such a marriage of "higher" and "lower" takes place, true unconditional love unfolds, embracing and penetrating all aspects of being, transforming the worldly into the Divine. Where there used to be judgment, there is now acceptance, combined with hightened faculties of perception and discrimination.

Negative emotions cannot prevail over love. Whenever you attend lovingly to your anger or despair, or sadness, feeling them fully, they quickly dissolve, as if vanished into thin air. Loving your illness also promotes healing. When you love your illness for the message or lesson it wants to convey to you, a healing quickly takes place.

By experiencing fully all your resistance and your desire for love and approval, and feeling gratitude for the instances of love you have been blessed to encounter in the course of your life, you will eventually open to the presence of unconditional love. Unconditional love is the highest form of abundance there is, and very healing, too, for love is the most life affirming quality there is.

# Step 5
## (Days 5, 12, and 19)

*Experience the thoughts
and resulting emotions
that block the flow of abundance
in the fifth or throat chakra*

Sit in a comfortable position, your spine erect, yet relaxed, your ears over your shoulders and your shoulders over your hips,
> *for 5 minutes*
> *feel your resistance to true communication.*

Experience fully, with complete *enthusiasm* how difficult it is for you to communicate your truth.

Recall certain incidents over the past week where you did not speak your truth, either by omission, or with a falsehood. Feel the result in the entire body and expand it until it dissipates.

Now,
    *for 5 minutes,*
    *feel your desire for true communication.*

Experience this desire fully, with complete *enthusiasm*. Feel how much you seek true communication. Feel fully how relieved you would be to finally speak your truth.

Think of specific examples of people to whom you would like to communicate your true feelings. Imagine yourself doing so. Now experience the resulting emotions throughout the entire body and expand until they dissipate.

Finally,
    *for 5 minutes*
    *consider all the instances in your life,*
    *when you were and will be able*
    *to communicate your truth.*

Experience gratitude for all your past, present and future experiences with true communication.

After you are complete, bring the attitude of gratitude into every communication. Let the attitude of gratitude touch you whenever you communicate your true feelings during the day.

# Commentary

All communication issues are particularly connected to blockages in this energy center, because it is in the throat, that sounds originate. The throat chakra has a function similar to a bridge; it links the head and body together, and enables you to use your voice to communicate your ideas and inner feelings.

In order to allow for an abundance of truth, you have to first deal with your resistance against true communication. Try to recall instances when you did not want to speak up, when you did not say what was moving through you, such as a feeling tone, an observation, a state of mind expressing who you were in that moment. Experience your resistance against your own truth. Experience your meek, evasive voice, your avoidance of eye contact. Notice the little lies that cross your mind.

Observe whom you are protecting. What are you hiding from the other? What are you trying to hide from yourself? You are not trying to make the resistance go away. You are not aiming for any preconceived, ready-made truth. For five minutes, just listen to your resistance against your inner voice.

In an ancient Indian prayer, the purity of truthful communication is expressed beautifully: " ...ether element, origin of heaven, transluscent, crystal-like, pure and without flaw, in such beauty and graceful motion radiates the world, like silver rays of moon dispelling darkness." When you experience communication as a gesture of Universal Life Force Energy, you are able to communicate the knowledge of the heart. Like "rays of moonlight", your communication dispels darkness. Since the knowledge of the heart is your very own truth, you communicate nothing but the truth.

True communication can only happen when you know how to listen. You can learn how to listen by attending to the habits and tendencies that prevent you from listening to your own inner voice. Once you are in contact with truth as your source, it is easy to speak it out appropriately, at the right time, and in the right way.

Communication is an important factor in manifesting abundance in the material realm. When we speak our intention from true Self, the Universe reacts. In the material realm, our abundance is also a direct result of our interplay with others. Although others can never be the source of our abundance (only true Self is this source), the relaxed ease with which we express and communicate the abundance we are to others, determines the ease and scope of its actual manifestation.

Therefore, by addressing our resistance, desire and gratitude for the ability to communicate truthfully, we open ourselves to a natural flow of abundance in our lives.

# Step 6
## (Days 6, 13, and 20)

*Experience the thoughts
and resulting emotions
that block the flow of abundance
in the sixth or "third eye" chakra*

Sit in a comfortable position, your spine erect, yet relaxed, your ears over your shoulders and your shoulders over your hips,
> *for 5 minutes*
> *contemplate your resistance*
> *to your inner knowing.*

Experience fully, with complete *enthusiasm* the difficulties you have trusting your intuition, and any fears that surface as a reaction to the guidance of your inner knowing.

Recall certain incidents where as an afterthought you later wished you had followed your first impulse. Experience the resulting emotions throughout the entire body and expand until they dissipate.

Now,
> *for 5 minutes,*
> *contemplate your desire for inner knowing.*

Experience this desire fully, with complete *enthusiasm*, feeling how much you want this inner knowing; how much you want to trust your intuition, and become one with it.

Experience this feeling throughout the entire body and expand until it dissipates.

Finally,
> *for 5 minutes*
> *cultivate the attitude of gratitude*
> *for all the instances in your life,*
> *when you were, are and will be*
> *a channel for all knowledge flowing through.*

Feel your gratitude for all your past, present and future experiences with inner knowing.

After you are complete, try to carry over this attitude of gratitude into the way you perceive things intutively.

# Commentary

All issues of intuition and inner knowing are particularly connected to this energy center, because it is through the so-called "third eye" that all the five senses combined with the "sixth sense" of awareness penetrate the "outer" and "inner" worlds. This chakra is the "wisdom eye" of inner knowing which evokes a more broad and continuous participation in life's unfolding. Such inner knowing embraces all aspects of life in a balanced manner.

Inner knowing, intuition, and conscious awareness are the seeds of manifestation. Therefore, this energy center has been linked since time immemorial to the capacity to manifest objects and events, even to the point of their materialization and/or dematrialization.

The energy of conscious awareness has the power to create new realities or to dissolve the structures supporting reality as we know it. It can suspend the laws of Newtonian physics.

The Sanskrit word for this energy center is *ajna*, which means "command and control". The more ordinary levels of reality, symbolized by the root, belly, solar plexus, heart, and throat chakras are controlled by and receive commands from the "third eye". Although generally associated with the pineal gland, this function of "command and control" is further stressed by the close connection between this energy center and the pituitary gland which also governs the endocrine system, which is also the physiological counterpart of the other chakras.

In this capacity of unlocking realms of experience "right here" that are, in any ordinary sense, "not in this time and space", an abundance of intuition and inner knowing points toward and expresses the inherent unity of all things in true Self. Therefore, the degree of intuition and inner knowing we enjoy shows how much we are in touch (or out of touch) with our true Nature, because the more we are in touch, the more knowledge can flow through and manifest through us.

One word to the wise, this process of opening to more and more knowledge flowing through us, cannot be controlled as in the ordinary approach of ego collecting, hoarding and manipulating information. Instead, it happens due to a sudden or gradual surrender to the knowledge which is already there. This surrender proceeds gently enough to naturally protect you against becoming overwhelmed by an overload of "telepathic" input. Intuition will reveal exactly what needs to be known in any given moment. Thus, you don't have to do anything, not even protect yourself.

Since intuition is always available, the only thing you need to "do" in order to unlock its potential, is to feel your resistance and desire for it and gratefully accept that which is already there for you. With this inherent ability that is your birthright, you can enjoy abundance by stretching and transcending the limits of what you have been programmed to conceive as real.

# Step 7
## (Days 7, 14, and 21)

*Experience the thoughts
and resulting emotions
that block the flow of abundance
in the seventh or crown chakra*

Sit in a comfortable position, your spine erect, yet relaxed, your ears over your shoulders and your shoulders over your hips,
*for 5 minutes*
*feel all of your resistance to true Self.*
Experience with complete *enthusiasm* how difficult it is for you to surrender to true Self. Feel how afraid you are to let true Self determine the course of your life.

Recall incidents where you really felt the need for Divine support, but because of your beliefs, you couldn't perceive it there, already inside of you. Experience your need throughout your entire body and expand it until it dissipates.

Now,
*for 5 minutes,*
*contemplate your desire for true Self.*
Experience this desire with complete *enthusiasm*, feeling fully how much you desire enlightenment; how much you want to become one with it.

Experience your tendency to seek greater knowledge or experience outside of yourself. Recall specific incidents and experience them throughout the entire body and expand until they dissipate.

Finally,
*for 5 minutes*
*cultivate the attitude of gratitude*
*for the enlightenment that you already are.*
Feel deeply grateful for all your past, present and future experiences of enlightenment.

After you are complete, you need not even try to carry over this attitude of gratitude into the way you live enlightenment every day of your boundless life. No longer perceiving anyone outside true Self to thank, just be.

# Commentary

All issues of enlightenment are particularly connected to this energy center, because it is in the so-called "crown chakra" where there is no form, only limitless and unmanifest Divine Being.

Nothing much can be said about enlightenment. On one occasion, the Buddha kept silent, smiled and showed a flower. Only one disciple got the message, and this was the origin of the Zen transmission.

Ultimately this perfect state has to be realized in the human heart, where the illusory ego is finally dissolved—where Enlightenment *is*—no mind, no thoughts.

One of my teachers once shared a wonderful story about a very rare man. This man without a mind and without thoughts decided one day to take a short nap under a tree. When he woke up an hour later and was about to continue on his lone journey, he saw himself surrounded by many gods and beings of light. They bowed before him and thanked him for his teaching. He didn't understand; with a baffled expression he said: "But I didn't even say one word. I was just napping. Why are you all here?"

"This may be so", one of the beings of light answered, "and yet we would have never received a teaching like this in our Divine realm. The countless distractions of the many pleasures in heaven and all the things we have to do demand our constant attention. For a change, we wanted to have some quiet and peace of mind, and found you. It was wonderful to be with you, because a man with no thoughts in his mind emits the energy of peace and love."

To *be* is a question of surrender to Being. Open space, nothing holy, but every little no-thing very sacred.

# Introduction To the 21-Day Plan To Complete Abundance

## Beginning the 21-Day Plan to Complete Abundance

In the course of the first 21 days, you have experienced how resistance and desire effect the important issues in our lives and how our reactions to these issues are reflected throughout the entire body-mind. By becoming aware of whatever resistance and desire you felt concerning these seven important areas of self-expression, you then completed each session by exploring your feelings of deep gratitude for the experiences you have had in your life. You may have even palpably sensed that both resistance and desire were simultaneously dissolved when touched by the attitude of gratitude. In the state of gratitude you were then able to experience the ever-presence of abundance where before you may only have felt lack.

Now, you can complete the final step. Over the next 21 days you will have the opportunity to open yourself to complete abundance. By directly accessing unity, you can achieve this almost miraculous shift from the ordinary mind set of lack, to the all-pervading abundance of the ocean of consciousness (or Universal Life Force Energy). By focusing all of your attention on the process, you will enable yourself to touch and even taste the underlying oneness inherent in your life.

We are human beings. We have a human body and mind with some incredible, even awesome abilities that, if acknowledged and used properly, empower us to fully be, to fully partake in the dance of Universal Life Force Energy. At heart, we are source and substance of true Self. True Self is nothing other than what we are, but it is *not the same* as what we usually

105

think we are. We have a choice. We can either continue to follow the messages, models, identifications and delusions that alienate us from the Source that we are, or we can dive right into Source and surrender to the refreshing waters of Life.

The following seven steps are not positive affirmations, or figments of imagination. Rather, they are statements of Reality as such. They evoke true Self, God-Self, primordial Being, Universal Life Force Energy, or whatever else you prefer to call this very Oneness that can even allow for the illusion of separation and duality to happen.

Although you can use these statements in different ways, they involve two elements you cannot change. First: You have to work with one of them each day for at least fifteen minutes. Second: You have to utilize them in three 7-day cycles for a total of 21 consecutive days. On the first day, you spend fifteen minutes on the first statement, on the second day you spend fifteen minutes on the second statement, and so on until, on the seventh day, the first cycle is complete. On day eight (day 29 of the entire 42-day program), you start the second cycle, and on day fifteen (day 36 of the entire 42-day program) the third. The three repetitions help to ground the truth of these statements *in your personal* reality. It is also recommended that you initially repeat the daily statement three times from Core Self, which helps make them *real for you.* There is an esoteric law which states that anything repeated three times will become truth.

Apart from these two ground rules, you are free to focus on the statements as you please: in a more formal style or rather informally; while sitting, standing or walking (but not laying down, because you will tend to become drowsy). Provided you concentrate on the subject at hand and not on the energy flow, you can even give yourself Reiki during the process (although self treatments will have far better results during this period of internal cleansing, if you do them separately, preferably in the evening).

For best results, a more formal approach to the statements might prove helpful. Remember that with these statements from Core-Self, you are counteracting millennia of negative conditioning that have kept you locked away in the limited consciousness of lack. You have the opportunity to turn your life around completely, from head to heart, and uncover the ever-presence of abundance that has remained hidden from you for a very long time. A little effortless concentration and a relaxed focus on what you are doing will go a long way. Therefore I suggest the following (or a similar) approach.

The ideal time for this plan, is in the morning before starting your day. This way, you re-program yourself before the outside world has a chance to do the job for you (for its own benefit *not* yours).

## Preparation for the Steps to Complete Abundance

Sit in a comfortable position either in a chair or on a cushion on the floor, your spine straight and relaxed, your ears over your shoulders and your shoulders over your hips. Now, bring your awareness to your breathing. Just watch your breath for a short while. Don't alter it. Don't do anything to it. Just continue breathing in and out naturally, effortlessly.

Appreciate the peace of sitting quietly. Appreciate being by yourself. Acknowledge how awake you are, how aware you are, how fresh you are in this moment. As you relax, your perception becomes as calm and as clear as the surface of a mountain lake. Feel your energy becoming focused as you turn your awareness to your intent. Bring your attention to your heart so that you become open and receptive enough to absorb the results. Know that the process will touch you and change the way you interpret the events in your life. The essence of who you are will not change, yet nothing will remain as it used to be, because you'll see it differently.

Now start with the process. Read today's statement and feel the meaning permeate your whole being while you internally repeat the words. Repeat the entire statement at least three times. Don't think! Allow yourself to be touched. Allow yourself to be uplifted. Allow yourself to experience the grace of Universal Life Force Energy directly addressing you. Truth is speaking to you. Self is speaking to you, gently awakening you to that which has been yours for eons, which has been your birthright since beginningless time. By considering the words of these Core Statements you are energetically exploring the reality they describe.

# A 21-Day Plan
# To
# Complete Abundance

# Statement 1
(day 22, 29, and 36)


The Universal Life Force Energy *I AM*
is the very source and substance
of *true SELF.*
It is who *I AM.*
My physical form is the fountain
through which the vibration of *true SELF* flows;
through which my whole universe manifests.
I turn now to that source of infinite prosperity,
which is the true source and substance of all.

# Commentary

Abundance is not something you find outside of yourself; it is a state of being that you experience in your mind. Through your trust in your innate ability to attract abundance you actually enable yourself to experience it in the outer world. To live in abundance, I have to remember and affirm my essence which is the very wellspring of my prosperity.

I need to remember that I am not my ego with its survivalist mentality, struggling to make a buck, or trying desperately to hang on to what I already have. I am much greater than that.

The first step to realizing abundance is to wake up to the fact that true Self, the Divine essence within us, is who we truly are. When we realize our source, it is then easy to surrender the false "self" to that greater power within us. By turning our awareness to true Self, and allowing ourselves to follow our hearts' desire, we soon realize that we have been *THAT* all along: simply as individualized vehicles of that very essence *I AM*.

With this awareness, true Self is then free to express openly in all our dealings with the outside world. In this state, I experience openness, emptiness, nothing-ness. Nobody home, only Self. It is not even that I turn toward Source, as Source is always there just resting in its infinite potential. It is simply that by turning my attention to the Infinite Source that *I AM*, I too am empowered to experience my infinite potential. I then move beyond the normal limitations of everyday existence, and open to a vast possibility of richness.

# Statement 2
## (Day 23, 30, and 37)

I now turn all "I" thoughts inward
to the one Universal Power that
is individualized as me.
I recognize that all ego driven "*I*" thoughts such as:
"*I* will do this."; "*I* have decided that.";
"*I* do not want this."; or "*I* want that." are mind games
which lead to more suffering,
because they separate me
from True Source or Self.
Therefore I turn now to Universal Life Force Energy
which *I AM -*
in total trust
to look after all my needs.

# Commentary

In the first statement, we declared the supremacy of Self which we then acknowledged. As Core Self we discover ourselves to be the source of infinite prosperity, the very substance of all there is. What could be more abundant than that very substance?

In the second step we recognize what is separating us from Source. We acknowledge how the old pattern of focusing on an "I" *separate* from Universal Source, first puts up partitions and boundaries that, although illusory, cut off our natural flow of energy. This same "I" which is constantly making plans and decisions (and never has enough) is incapable of granting true abundance. Abundance and cutting off the natural flow are mutually exclusive. Every want I voice implies that I don't have. For true abundance to manifest the cutting off of Source has to cease.

With new found trust, I am now able to voice my needs, knowing without doubt that they will be provided, as Universal Source is who *I AM*.

Turning within, I drop all thoughts of separation and turn toward the Universal Power which *I AM*—which is responsible for all manifestation, which is responsible for giving light to the sun, which is responsible for giving power to the earth, to look after all my needs.

# Statement 3

### (Day 24, 31, and 38)

I accept all heartfelt desires to be
 Divine Universal Source
working through me, guiding me
toward the fruition of my task on this earth.
Therefore "I" let go,
and allow this Universal Source
to work through "me".
Not getting attached to these desires,
I surrender gratefully to Universal Life Force Energy
flowing through me,
lovingly accepting all the abundance
which is my true state.

# Commentary

In truth, desires are neither good nor bad. They are simply the vehicles which guide us toward fulfilling our roles in the world. Desire serves an important purpose. It is essential, as it acts as a guiding impulse to take us where we need to go.

If we rid ourselves of all desire, how could we ever accomplish what we originally set out to do when we were born on the earth in this particular role? Our desires are our guiding light. Desires lead us to the people and places we need to meet and experience, in order to learn the lessons we came here to learn. How could you become a doctor, if you didn't have a desire to become one in the first place? Without the desire for love, how could we connect with others or with Core Self? If it were not for the Universe's desire for growth and evolution, would each of us ever grow and mature?

Perhaps the best way to approach our desires, is to simply enjoy their unfolding; to let them be and let them go. In order to learn the lessons of our desires, it is best not to get hooked, but to let them flow through our experience by remaining unattached. Instead, you can accept all *heartfelt* desires as Divine Universal Source working through you. Like need that turns into neediness when unacknowledged, desires turn into a trap only when repressed or misused to support false identities. It is therefore wise to surrender all attachments to your role in life, and simply allow the desires of your role to play themselves out.

Eventually you begin to understand what Shakespeare also understood: "All the world's a stage and all the men and women merely players." We are here to play our role. The key is not to be identified with it. Ultimately you cannot explain or understand Life, you can only experience it and knowingly participate in its mysteries.

# Statement 4
### (Day 25, 32, and 39)

In my everyday activities I fully relinquish
my previous attachment to the "doer" or the "doing".
I now allow all activities to flow from Source,
that calm, centered state of Being that *I AM*.
My life is now unimpinged with any resistance due
to my prior mental habit of attachment to results.
Due to this shift in awareness,
all my activities now flow in a
well-balanced, *GRACEful* manner,
allowing even greater abundance to flow through me.

# Commentary

Everyone has at one time or another experienced the accomplishment resulting from free flowing activity. Things just seem to happen with total synchronicity. You don't waste any thought on who is doing it. Actually, you don't waste any thought at all, not even on the doing. It is a paradox, a complete mystery. On the one hand it feels as if you are involved in what you are doing, on the other hand, you are detached, almost not there, as if awareness is doing "it" for you.

In some spiritual traditions this is called "doing without doing" and considered a sign of realization. Rather than being an achievement it simply *is*: an expression of the natural state of Being which manifests the moment we let go of all the "hooks" (whatever we are attached to or identify with).

The calm, centered state of *I AM* could be compared to the screen in a movie theater. The screen has no investment in the pictures. It just allows them to move across its surface. However, when the pictures come to an end, the screen remains. Therefore, the all-encompassing screen represents a far greater state of abundance than the pictures that are by nature limited.

It is wise to be like the screen which does not get emotionally hooked by the experiences moving across it. It remains the same empty screen no matter what pictures or circumstances seem to be encompassing it. Similarly, if you just allow the events of your life to flow through you unencumbered, you'll enjoy a sense of freedom and abundance that embraces everything there is.

Deep inside you know this to be true. You have tasted freedom at least once in your life (if not, you would not have bothered to buy this book). You remember the special times when everything fell into place, when you were totally present, yet strangely uninvolved. You remember that you were neither smug nor arrogant, nor disinterested. Quite the contrary, the well-balanced, graceful manner of unfolding you experienced was the unconditional love we all contact when we let go of being the doer, and all the doing, and allow ourselves to simply *be*.

# Statement 5

(Day 26, 33, and 40)

As I constantly turn inward
to the Divine Source of my abundance
I discover through deeper self inquiry
that the various masks of "I" do not exist;
that when I ask myself in all earnestness:
"Who am *I*?",
I experience silence.
I experience a state of silence which reveals
the truth of the no-thing that *I AM*,
for *I AM* the nothing through which *everything* flows.

# Commentary

*I AM* the vast ocean of consciousness who once thought "I" was a wave, separate from other "waves" and not a part of this very same ocean that *I AM*.

As this realization dawns in your awareness, it is easy to relinquish all worries as a total waste of time and energy. As your faith and knowledge in the Divine Source of boundless *I AM* increases, the concerns that used to block your flow of abundance are swallowed in the wake of your deepening trust.

It is all so simple and so easy, hard to believe how you could ever convince yourself otherwise. When, you disengage from attachment to your beliefs and let go of what limits you, the resulting awareness reveals your true nature. Liberated from the heavy load of false identities you can then deeply ask that burning question: "Who am I?" As a consequence of the silence which results when this question is asked, you discover experientially that you are not any one particular thing, item or entity, but much, much vaster. You are limitless, and since you are not defined by any boundaries, everything can flow through you, manifest through you. The farther your letting go extends into the realm of timeless and spaceless Reality, the deeper the joy.

Your responsibilities are easily taken care of. Self now serves other beings as Self. There is no more confusion. Intuition sits in the driver's seat. Spontaneous knowing functions through your mind and brain, and it does a much better job than the false identity that used to pretend to run the show for you. You have now switched from "man-power" to Divine Power.

# Statement 6
### (Day 27, 34, 41)

Knowing from Source
that anger is merely an expression of
my being identified with past judgments
and dependent on my attachment to results,
I now allow myself to feel it fully and let it go.

## *Commentary*

In this statement, true Self expresses the paradox involved in liberating yourself from fruitless emotionality. The trick to freeing yourself from emotions is neither to control and suppress them nor to act them out. Controlling or repressing them hardens you, makes you passive-aggressive and eventually even physically sick. Acting them out just fuels the fire of emotionality, limiting what you can perceive of the whole of Reality. Instead of following either one of these options, you can now consciously choose to experience all of your emotions fully. By feeling them fully you move through and come out on the other side, which is the bliss of unconditional love.

As I come increasingly in contact with true Self, I recognize that all anger happens when I am still identified with the little "I" which has attachments to results either regarding a situation, or from another individual, when things don't go my way.

I do not resist this anger, but instead choose to feel it fully, with complete *enthusiasm* until it reveals its own source—the little "I" or ego that is still attached to some result. With my new willingness to experience my anger fully, my desire to act it out on another decreases. I begin to see that the "other" (person) is never the real cause of my anger.

With this increased awareness, I easily give up my need to control others. I cease projecting my anger out on "them", and less and less bounces back on me, as I also no longer attract others who project their anger onto me. The resulting blissful surrender to true Self, which brings an abundance of joy and peace, compensates one hundred fold for the giving up of a controlled and controlling ego.

# Statement 7
### (Day 28, 35 and 42)

Through my awareness
of Universal Life Force Energy
as the Source and supply of all my needs,
I show gratitude to every living thing
in all my words and actions,
accepting graciously from all others, as well as giving.
With no specific expectations
I now recognize all "others"
as fellow channels of abundance
like so many more waves in the
ocean of consciousness
with as much true Self as *I AM.*

# Commentary

We have been conditioned to rely on our egos and to depend on specific people or circumstances to provide our needs. The inherent limitations in such "providers" also limits the provisions they are fit to grant. When you subscribe to the limited beliefs and resources you were trained to believe in by your conditioning, you consciously or unconsciously limit the unlimited. If you want to live in abundance you have to be open to all possibilities. You have to categorically stop expecting anything from any one particular source, whether that be your job, a person, or a situation.

Instead, through your awareness of Universal Life Force Energy, you see and experience all outer "sources" as the one True Source. Being other waves on the ocean of consciousness, they, too, are channels of true abundance. Remember also, that expectations which are charged with emotion can create resistance and in turn block the flow of abundance, which would otherwise make itself obvious in a vast number of wonderful and surprising ways. It is better to know and trust that what is yours will be provided to you at just the right time and in a proper manner.

In short, the way of abundance is the way of receptivity and joyous acceptance. You accept the fact that you are not what you think you are, but what you intuitively *feel* you are. You are like an all-encompassing vessel. You are not *in* your body, your body is inside of You. Since you are all-encompassing, everything can come to you. Allow this to be your reality, and Reality will reward you.

Gentle and allowing, you thank every living thing in word and action, knowing it to be true Self. You totally live in the attitude of gratitude. No error is possible, even seemingly adverse circumstances turn into blessings. When trusting true Self and surrendering to Universal Life Force Energy, you cannot go astray. You are already there.

# Chapter 5

# Experiences With The 42-Day Abundance Program

The 42-day program to absolute fulfillment enables you to combine both the male aspect of the active pursuit of happiness and a more female joyous acceptance of what already is through the power and wisdom of Core Self. Once you have completed the program, you will be much more in touch with your inner knowing that actually there is only *one* Self and that you and all beings and appearances *are* this one Self. During the course of the second 21-day plan the process of direct self-inquiry helped you to realize the truth of I AM THAT which accommodates and perceives everything, and yet at the same time remains free of everything.

This powerful I AM is not the same as the ego or personality that you believe you are. Rather it is the incomprehensible silence you experience whenever you ask yourself the question: "Who am I?" Whenever you delve deep into this question with all your heart and energy, you finally penetrate THAT, the I AM which is the silent background or screen on which the play of life unfolds.

The paradox is that you will be more fulfilled in your ordinary everyday existence the more you open to the true Self that you are, while at the same time dissolving your identification with all of the "positive" *or* "negative" roles and experiences that you *appear to be*. Once you open to true Self, everything will flow through. The roles that you came into this life to experience, and the experiences you have attracted to learn from will make you richer, because you will *not* get hooked; they'll make you happy, because you will *not* get attached;

and they'll set you free, because you will *not* feel identified with them. You will be free and at peace to *be*.

The four accounts in this chapter were written by students who have completed the 42-day program after attending the *Core Abundance Seminar*. They give a fairly good idea of the many concrete results that can be experienced through this approach.

A closer look also shows that all these results are not so much an end in themselves but rather enriching and liberating stages on an open ended journey. This journey beckons you further and further, ever deeper into abundance. Of course, names and particular circumstances have been changed to protect the privacy of the students.

As my awareness expands,
my range of possibilities in the outer world also expands.
I gradually develop a larger sphere of influence
and an abundance of everything
I am now open to
naturally flows toward me.

# The Core Abundance Seminar

To facilitate a quick approach to the processes of the 42-day program, the *Core Abundance Seminar* is offered as a powerful one day program. It is designed to help each individual experience his or her own true identity and potential as it goes right into the core of personal abundance issues.

As stated before: Abundance is not so much a question of how much or how little you have, but rather an expression of how complete you feel with yourself. By introducing you to the real *limitless you*, the *Core Abundance Seminar* promotes a clean break with thousands of years of unhealthy identification with scarcity and never ending neediness. During the course of this powerful day, participants learn to see themselves as the source of their fulfillment. In the morning session, we explore the belief patterns which keep people from fulfilling their heartfelt desires. By the afternoon, participants are introduced to the process of how to manifest abundance in their lives.

A lot of tears and laughter are shared as we discover both the grievous sabotage we have done to ourselves and the ridiculously funny beliefs we have bought into, which have kept us from experiencing our true state of abundance. I share a lot of my own silly experiences as well, as they seem to have helped many of my students integrate in a very short time what may have taken me months or years to learn. However, participation in the seminar is not a prerequisite for your successful work with the 42-day program. Like yourself, the participants have to eventually delve deeply into the 42-day process in order to realize through direct self-inquiry what is already theirs. The seminar serves as an introduction, it is not a short-cut.

## Robert:
## One Surprise After The Other

"I practiced an early version of the 42-day program and had many experiences which took me by surprise even though I had previously worked with some of Paula's material.

When I started the program I had no expectations. I was interested and wanted to give it the effort it deserved. But I didn't think it would trigger extraordinary results or set in motion such unexpected developments.

Every morning in the course of the first 21-day plan I became aware of patterns that I had never seen before with the same sense of clarity. This is strange, I thought, here I am, a successful business man and successful Reiki master, teacher of a variety of consciousness techniques—and still hooked on stereotypes and restrictive behaviour?

127

For example, I realized that despite all my successes I still shied away from all-out success, because I didn't want to hurt my father who had also been a successful business man in his own right, but never managed to reach the high goals he had set for himself. I got in touch with the sense that unconsciously it didn't feel right to better my old man. Other patterns also became obvious; my need to be helpful, my obsessive seeking, and so forth. Everything became clear in a very fresh and spontaneous way. After a few days I was actually looking forward to the sessions, and I also most often took more time than the fifteen minutes suggested in the introduction. I was never disappointed.

After the 42 days were over, I felt lighter, freer and more alive. I had learned quite a bit about myself and made some progress on the path to greater awareness. As far as I was concerned, the program had already given me more than I had expected to receive.

Then, one morning about two weeks later, I received a telephone call. The assistant to a TV producer called me up and asked me if I would like to be interviewed for a one hour special on Reiki. She cautioned me not to expect too much. There would be other Reiki masters, and there would be expert opinions by medical doctors. As a matter of fact the first meeting would just be about getting to know each other and finding out if I would be comfortable on TV. Would I want to give it a try? Without wasting much thought I said yes.

On the morning of the actual meeting with the producer and director of the show, I sat down to go through the process of resistance, desire and gratitude. I first went into my resistance against showing off, then into my desire for sharing my experiences with Reiki and finally into the feeling of gratitude for the opportunity that had manifested of its own accord. It took almost half an hour before I was through. Afterwards I felt open, and didn't even think about the meeting and what to say.

Everything worked out much better than I could ever have

expected in my wildest dreams. When we sat down to talk I didn't even try to prove anything, I didn't attempt to sell Reiki, I just shared my truth and my experiences. The conversation became more and more lively, and I totally forgot that the purpose was to determine if I was fit for appearing on TV. However, to my surprise in the end I was picked not only to do the show, but they also asked if I would be willing to do a more comprehensive program where I would be the only guest. So I had my thirty minutes on the screen and was able to share my views. It was a great boost for my activities."

## Valerie:
## Dropping Trauma-Identity

"I have been in therapy for several years to heal the wounds of a traumatic childhood experience. Despite all the time I have taken to deal with this issue, it has been very difficult to let go of it. I still felt identified with the trauma I'd undergone, despite all the progress I'd made in detaching myself from this memory. Until very recently it has been really hard for me to drop the negative mental tape that has kept me bound to something I have deeply resented all my life.

Several months ago a friend suggested that I take the *Core Abundance Seminar* as a playful way to engage my desire to be fulfilled and whole, and to help release this negative memory. The seminar itself was a wonderful experience. Everybody got into the partner exercises with great enthusiasm. The talks on the different issues related to abundance were very lively, and some of the interactions in the group inspired me a lot, because they mirrored things that I had not noticed yet myself. When I left the seminar room I felt great, even a little elated.

On the second day of my 42-day program, crisis hit. I was shocked when I read the instruction. I vehemently resisted the idea of being grateful for my negative sexual experiences. This was asking too much of me. But I forced myself to do the exercise, because the seminar had been so inspiring. I really wanted to trust the process and find out if it would really work. Strong emotions that I thought I had put behind me rose to the surface.

I remembered all the years of therapy, when I had tried to accept and feel my rage against the man who had raped me when I was a child. When I finally had crossed the threshold of fear, I had screamed and cried many times until I could scream and rage no more, ...and now I was asked to be thankful for this negative sexual experience!

After the exercise I felt restless to the point that I began to obsess on the of thought how much this exercise reminded me of rape. Had it not forced me to think thoughts that I didn't want to think, that went totally against my feelings? I felt abused. The memory of the experience had again felt much too close. At one point I couldn't stand feeling lost and helpless, confronted with old memories that were too much for me to handle.

Finally I gave Paula a call. We only talked for a few minutes, and what I remembered from the conversation was her insisting that with feeling grateful for all the experiences in my life, both negative and positive, I would be able to take back my power. This was exactly what I wanted. I did not wish to continue to define my whole life through the focus of this hideous experience from the past. Furthermore, she explained to me that it was not so much a case of feeling gratitude for the actual experience of abuse as it was for the final *lesson* of the experience. She helped me realize that if I continued to interpret the experience as a reflection of me not being good enough, or if I continued to interpret it in such a way that I made myself a victim, I would stay a victim.

I decided to follow through with all the steps of the 42-day program. I didn't notice any other dramatic shifts except the letting go of this old tape. It really feels like I've finally let go. I also have the sense that from now on my past will not continue to define my present."

This story illustrates the powerful effect of the first 21-day plan while working with resistance, desire and gratitude. Provided you get as involved with the process, with as much strong intention as Valerie did, and allow yourself to feel your feelings fully, you will experience a deep letting go. Your feelings of resistance, desire and gratitude will dissolve your tendency to identify with the terrible experiences and tragedies which may have happened to you earlier in your life. You will no longer feel victimized, even if you have previously felt consumed by the victim role.

Having been sexually abused as a young girl, Valerie understandably resisted feeling gratitude for this abuse. However, I was able to point out to her that she was not asked to be grateful for the abuse itself, but for the *role* it had played in her life. Tragic as it had been, the abuse was also the driving force behind her yearning for conscious awareness. Through her deep self-work she had become a very mature woman.

If a person who has been physically or psychologically abused continues to interpret the experience as a reflection of their not being good enough or as a victim, he or she will continue to perpetuate the suffering inherent in this role. Gratitude helps to take us beyond this vicious circle. By cultivating gratitude for every moment of her life, Valerie took back her life and her power.

Another thought which is also worth considering is that if at some point after processing our own pain we also allow ourselves to experience fully the pain of the person who inflicted the abuse, we get in touch with the abuse they also suffered. This helps us to finally get to the point where we don't take the abuse personally. Knowing that no one would abuse another if they themselves had not not already been abused, we break the chain of abuse at a very deep level and empower our lives even further.

# Carl:
## To Be Vulnerable Is To Be Strong

"I used to be an air force officer. When I was younger I flew fighter air craft and ended my career as a Colonel. Since my recent retirement, I've had a difficult time trying to find another job to keep myself busy. My wife is still working full time managing a large office. With all the time I have on my hands I began to notice how much I miss my wife. For years, she was always telling me how much she missed me, and now when the tables had turned, I felt very rejected. I really wanted to deepen my relationship with her, but it seemed that whatever I did, it just pushed her further away.

The day I joined the *Core Abundance Seminar*, I was deeply immersed in these and similar thoughts and feelings. The setting did little to alleviate my doubts. What good would it do to spend a whole day in a luxury five-star hotel, with a large group of people litening to a series of empty talks? Fortunately, my experience both during and after the seminar proved my expectations wrong.

During the partner exercises in the morning all my fears and judgments came up. I couldn't evade them. My eyes turned watery although I tried to hold back my tears and choke down my emotions. Out of the blue I heard my name and was instructed to sit across from my wife. I was then instructed to tell her what I needed. First I remained silent or could only speak a few words. Soon, however, the dam broke and all the things I had held back for so long spilled out. Although it seemed to take forever, it actually only took a few minutes, finally admitting to myself and to my wife how much I needed her.

It made me feel vulnerable to say that, but not weak. Quite the contrary, I really got how much strength there is in vulnerability. This was a deep realization for me. Like other men of my generation I had carried this false image of strength and independence. Later, during the 42-day program I went even deeper into exploring all the ramifications of this image. I was able to feel how much it had cut me off from the source of my abundance in relationship.

Now I understand that I never really had any problems with my wife. Due to my conditioning I had just bought into certain beliefs that convinced me of the reality of some imagined "problems". At this point, none of my daily circumstances have actually changed, and yet my life flows much more smoothly. My wife and I enjoy living and sharing together, both aware of how rich our lives actually always are. This is what I call bliss."


## Susan:
## An Obstacle Course Of Unconscious Desires

"Several weeks after I had completed my 42-day program I received the offer every real estate agent dreams of. If the deal was concluded, I wouldn't have to worry for the rest of my life. If at all, I could work for fun, simply because I like to be with people.

A wealthy developer was considering putting me in charge of all sales and leases for several new office buildings downtown. Considering the rapid growth of our city, it would be a foolproof opportunity, especially since high-tech companies from abroad seem to flock here no matter how much it will cost them.

There were a series of preliminary talks which all concluded on a harmonious note. With every additional meeting, my future partner appeared more courteous and agreeable. I didn't want to seem stand offish, so I became more charming myself, staying strictly within the limits of friendly business relations. If everything continued as it had started, we would soon be ready to sign a contract that would make me very rich. This idea seemed more and more appealing.

One week later we met for dinner without our associates. When the meeting was originally set up, I had felt uneasy for a few seconds, but I disregarded those feelings. Everything had gone well so far, and besides, I was sure that I had not given any signal that could be misinterpreted. I had actually been looking forward to the evening in one of the best restaurants in town. Over dessert the bombshell exploded. This man uttered in a pleasant voice and with a big smile on his face that he would very much like to sleep with me, as a matter of fact, he said we would be great lovers—as great as in business. The real threat remained unspoken, although it was clearly hanging in the air: no sex, no deal. Make up your mind girl.

That evening I managed to extricate myself with a lot of smiles and promising looks from a very tricky situation. When I finally reached home I felt like vomiting. All at once I felt anger, hurt and total despair. My old lack of self-confidence welled up. Why do women have to always put up with this kind of harrassment? Why are we objects of desire, and not appreciated for our talent or what we can achieve? It made me sick. I felt victimized and wallowed in self pity.

The following day I instructed my secretary not put any calls through to me from him or his office. One week later we had another meeting, but now it was mentioned that I would have to share this lucrative contract with several other real estate agents. I immediately interpreted the change as punishment for my being "un-cooperative", especially because new bribes for my "cooperation" seemed to be implicitly offered. Or was I simply paranoid?

At this point I decided to use this muddled situation to take a look at my whole life. I was lucky. Paula was in town for ten days, so I decided to register for her five day intensive, *The Core Empowerment Training*. It promises that "nothing will remain repressed, nothing unacknowledged" -that sounded just right for me.

It was not easy to discuss the problem in front of everybody in the group. I waited until the last day, to the last possible moment, until the inner pressure had built up and I couldn't possibly hold back any longer. When I spoke, many things became evident.

My whole life was on display, not only the "problem" at hand. I was determined not to feel victimized any more. I needed to reclaim my freedom of action. Thus I asked myself: how did I contribute to the situation? I immediately saw the part that I had repressed and denied in myself: my strong female sexuality. I am an attractive woman. I love life and all that it has to offer. I am successful, and success has sex-appeal. Nevertheless I had been living for years almost like a nun, mainly because after my share of disappointments in relationship, I had become overcautious—and perhaps also because I haven't allowed myself an abundance of feeling or expression.

What I came to realize is that if I deny my physical desires, my body will send out implicitly sexual signals, because my body always shows what my body needs. My prospective business partner had received those signals and interpreted them according to his own desires. I am not saying this in order to excuse his behaviour. It is totally disgusting to misuse power or any other kind of leverage for gaining sexual favors from others. On the other hand, I should have been consciously aware of my own desires instead of repressing them, in which case the whole muddled situation would not have occured. This is something I know from experience: When I am totally clear about myself, the other is equally clear about how far he can go. What Paula reminded me was that we can perceive each others bottom line instinctively.

At this point I regard the whole story as a learning experience. What I came to realize, is that life may even have something better in store for me, and as a result I have dropped my attachment to the potentially biggest deal of my entire career. I have also learned to accept my sexual desires, and I know that I will eventually fulfill them with the man of my choice.

When Paula confronted my pattern of avoidance she also suggested that I speak my word and let this man know in no uncertain terms that I was still the best person he could do business with but to energetically let him know that I was otherwise unavailable. I took the challenge. At this point I cannot say what the consquences will be. In any event, clearing the air made me feel better.

If I think back, the whole process started when I first did the 42-day program. My new openness had then attracted a potentially very appealing real estate deal to me. But I sabotaged my chance for quick success, because I became *attached* to the idea of this deal and also for years had denied appropriate expression to my feelings. On the other hand this whole unfolding of events taught me a lot about myself. Now I know beyond the slightest doubt that I need fulfillment in my private life as much as I need business success."

Chapter 6

# Nine Steps to Manifestation

## 1. *Commit to your heart's desire*

The first step to manifesting the people, circumstances or material requirements that you need in your life, is to get in touch with your deepest heartfelt desires. Instead of distracting yourself with illusory hopes and wishful thoughts, or working toward goals which are set out of a false sense of duty, it is essential to get in touch with what evokes a truly passionate response in your being. What is it that moves you at a heart level? What would you absolutely want to accomplish, if you had only one year to live? Only one week?

Unfortunately too many of us waste our entire lives deliberating about a variety of experiences we might engage in "one day". Instead of making a choice and putting our energy behind a firm decision, we waste a huge amount of time stuck in an uninspiring state of ambivalence. Waffling between desire and resistance, we often find it virtually impossible to get out of our head and into contact with our deepest heartfelt need.

To break this pattern there has to be a willingness to:
1. *Feel* your need.
2. *Decide* how to fulfill it.
3. *Commit* to make it happen.

To get in touch with what will truly fulfill you, it may be necessary to spend some quiet time with yourself and actually put your hands on your heart and ask what it needs. You might even give Reiki to your heart at the same time. So often we get lost in our heads and forget to give ourselves the time to recharge and nurture our inner child. The inner child is very

137

clear and knows just what it wants (and needs), if we will only listen.

Quite often our deepest desires do not match with our preconceived notions of what we think we "should" want. In actual fact, it would be very advisable to eliminate the word "should" from your vocabulary. It automatically infers someone or something outside of yourself is projecting a need or desire on you. The most common example is all the internal shoulds we carry which were ingrained in us by our parents, teachers and family. Once we unburden ourselves of all the shoulds, it becomes much easier to decide on a course of action. By making a firm decision, energetically we create a charge which sets all sorts of things in motion.

Our decision acts as a magnet which attracts all the circumstances we need, to create the reality we are seeking. By also eliminating the word "try" from our vocabulary, our actions are no longer sabotaged by a lukewarm commitment to our goals. Whenever we commit ourselves to any course of action, when we decide to do something (rather than try), we stand a far better chance of fulfilling our heartfelt desires.

What is helpful is to acknowledge your strongest desires as Universal will flowing through you, urging you to become more truly who you are. These desires are the lifeblood of our experience; the one's we intuitively feel will lead us to the circumstances we need to go through, in order to learn our greatest lessons and fulfill our tasks on the earth.

## 2. Set priorities

After getting in touch with the desire or few desires which really move you, it is important to decide on a course of action to bring them into reality. By envisioning clearly the preparations which are needed to realize your goals, you take a powerful step toward their final manifestation. Any choice which is not accompanied by a clear commitment to taking the necessary steps for its achievement, remains nothing but a fantasy, *and that fantasy will drain your psychic and creative energy faster than you realize.* Once you are set on your priorities, a clear commitment to take any necessary steps will help dissipate your desire and resistance.

Sometimes the steps you need to take will be quite obvious, at other times you may only be aware of one or two. Often with a new project, the first step is simply research. By commiting yourself to one or two choices and then actually pursuing them physically, you will cause later steps to reveal themselves of their own accord.

## 3. Envision your goal

In many of the ancient spiritual traditions, different exercises utilizing visualization were introduced to help each initiate learn to focus the mind. Various techniques were designed specifically to quiet the mind, as a mind which is constantly distracted by all the various circumstances flowing around it can never be one pointed. It will stand little chance of experiencing the blissful silence of no-mind which enables all things to flow through (including abundance)

On a more mundane level, visualization is a very powerful tool when you want to manifest certain goals. Earlier in the book, I shared about the experiences of one of my Australian students who, for five years, kept a very specific goal book, complete with clear visual photographs of exactly what she envisioned for herself. By being very specific about her goals, and daily, spending a certain amount of time visualizing them, she successfully achieved her goals in a relatively short amount of time.

Often it is helpful to write a specific list of what it is you want, and then cut out pictures from magazines or other sources which help illustrate what you intend to eventually manifest. Clear visualization helps concentrate energy and bring it into the realm of matter. For those who are not "naturally" visual, know that with practice all things are possible. It just may take further effort. If you are more kinesthetically inclined, you can always sense the presence of what it is you wish to manifest.

## 4. Love what you choose

*with full-bodied enthusiasm.*

It is absolutely essential to love what you do, and to cultivate full-bodied enthusiasm or ecstasy in all aspects of your life. Love and enthusiasm enable you to transmute through all of the various levels of emotion.

To experience abundance you have to be free of all your emotions about money and survival. During the 42-day program for *Core Abundance* you were able to concentrate on all of your emotional issues about abundance. By focusing your entire attention on your feelings, you successfully dissipated many old patterns, and became aware of the ones you may have previously taken for granted as fact. To further facilitate the flow of abundance, it is essential to imbue all of your heartfelt desires with love.

When you love what you do, you put your energy behind your bliss. Love energy is the energy of the universe. If you love what you do, the universe will surely be with you every step of the way. It is important to enjoy the process of working toward your goals, as it takes only a second to reach a goal, it generally takes weeks, months or even years to actually get there. A goal is always in the future, one step ahead of you, but life itself only takes place in the eternal moment. There is only one now..., now..., now..., and now, like pearls on a circular string, seemingly one now ofter the other, but truly just one long, infinite moment to be enjoyed.

# 5. Be in gratitude

Realize that what you desire in your heart, is already yours, it simply hasn't manifested in material reality, yet. By focusing on the attitude of gratitude for what you already have and for what you are going to have, you will continue to stay in the state of "have". It is essential to be in gratitude before you have even received the fulfillment of your desires, as a thankful heart is an open heart, and is thus open to receiving.

Also, by being grateful for what you already have, you further keep your *mind* in the state of have. Our entire experience of reality is a direct result of every thought we think. If you think lack you will receive lack. On the other hand, if you manage to keep your attention on abundance, you will most definitely experience more abundance.

To be in gratitude is to know at the core of your being that all is one, that separation is an illusion. Gratitude chips away at the illusion of separation as it tends to take you away from your focus on "self" or ego. As you are the center of your own universe it is easy to understand how ego begins to identify with all the experiences flowing through it, as if *it* is doing it. Whenever you say "Thank you", you naturally shift the focus away from the ego and its habit of taking credit, and include another. When things are going well, and especially if I am *not* satisfied in a situation, I say thank you to the power of love or to the energy flowing through me, to the people who channel abundance to me, to the fact that I can channel energy for myself or others. I say thank you to whatever comes to me.

When you practice gratitude in your life, the wonderment you once experienced as a child will gradually return to you. It is this childlike sense of awe, when accompanied by the wisdom of the adult, which helps imbue in us the state of non-causal joy which remains no matter how challenging life becomes.

## 6. Be willing to receive what is meant for you

One of the most important steps in the process of manifestation is the willingness to receive all of what life has to offer. Unfortunately, one of the most common beliefs people have deeply buried in the subconscious, is a feeling of unworthiness. Even people who are very successful in their lives, often become this way just to make themselves feel worthy. They often develop the "I'll do it myself" syndrome, and find it very difficult to receive from others. Often, this type needs to prove others wrong to make themselves right. This leads to a sense of struggle in life, as there is no easy give and take.

Through my many years of leading emotional release workshops, I have been amazed at how universal this deep sense of not being worthy of love is. When we don't feel worthy, we tend to use all sorts of means to get attention from others and to prove that we are "good enough".

"I'm not good enough", is one belief that we all need to feel fully and let go of. Every person on this earth is worthy of love. A deep sense of unworthiness is just what creates a Hitler or a Stalin. These two and many other minor versions of them, for the most part came into existence through severe mistreatment as children. Alice Miller's later books decry the harsh childhood of these abusive types and of man's inhumanity to children.

The examples I've given are extreme, but each one of us has at one time or another harboured a feeling of unworthiness. To help open your receiving channel, you need to get out of your head and focus on your heart. You might once again, put your hand on your heart and feel all your desire and resistance to receiving love. The fourth step in the first 21-day plan will also help you deal with this issue. Ultimately, you should have no doubt in your mind that you are worthy of abundance. Accept that you are worthy. Receive all that is meant for you with a grateful heart, and you will be richly rewarded.

# 7. Make it so with your word

Once you have commited to a firm decision and imbued it with love and gratitude, it is important to make it so with your word. Knowing clearly that you have done your utmost to energize whatever it is you choose to manifest, you can then declare that it is done. The simple statement "Make it so", or a precise statement of intent made in present tense, are appropriate at this point. Rather than saying: "I *will* do such and such" or "I *want* to have such and such", you say: "My project *is complete* on such and such date." It is important to go inside and feel (using your intuition) when you will realistically be able to manifest what you desire, and then set your date. It is best to focus on goals which can be completed within a one or two year period. If you have a long range goal, you can always put the intermediary steps you'll need to take into goal statements, which will then further charge your intention with energy. When you speak your goals from your heart, notice how you feel. If doubts come up allow yourself to feel them until they dissipate, and then make your statement again until you are absolutely sure that you are speaking your truth with total clarity.

It is best not to share your plans (or make your declarations of intent) with others of a negative mindset. Most people have a lot of "Yes, buts" floating around in their heads or thoughts like: "He or she will never do that". Such thoughts will dissipate the energy you are building up to manifest your project. I usually wait until I have laid a firm foundation for a new project, before I share it with others.

Once you have spoken your word, stick to it. So many people will tell you "I'll do this" or "I'll do that" and then do not follow through. Whenever you do not take action on your spoken word, you weaken yourself and strip yourself of power. We do it all the time in so many little ways. We make many seemingly small commitments to others which we then forget and do not follow through on. It is better to say no to others if you are not sure that you can comply; and especially in the case of a personal goal, you should not even state it, if you are not absolutely sure that you can complete it.

There is tremendous power in the spoken word when it comes from the heart of your truth. You charge yourself with faith and trust in the universe and really "make it so". When you use your word to establish your commitment, you also create a magnetic effect in the energy around you, which then draws to you whatever you need to manifest your abundance.

## 8. Take action

Once you have given your word to yourself (or others), it is important to follow up with action. Your action further charges the energy around you with your intention and helps to draw in the needed pieces of your puzzle. The greater your sense of separation from true Self, the greater your action is going to have to be in order to manifest.

A sense of relief will set in as soon as you begin to take action and notice your steady progress. This will help you relax so that you can open to insights which will also further support you in your process.

## 9. Surrender to true Self

Once we begin to take action, it is very easy for the ego to again get hooked to being the doer. You can manifest to a certain point when coming from ego, as is evident when you observe the world today. What is also obvious though, is that as long as ego is running the show, there is no sense of peace, and we fall right back into the trap of the survival game with its deep fear of lack. The victim role is also bound to set in again, and we then experience a repeat performance of the spiral downward into the illusion of "never enough".

The easy answer is to simply "let go and let God", as the old saying goes. Now that you have fully energized your intention by visualizing it, embuing it with love, expressing your gratitude, and taking action, what is left to do, is to simply let go of your attachment to your plan, and trust that the most perfect result will happen for the highest and best good. In effect, you now surrender "self" or ego to true Self—the Divine Abundant Self which is common to us all.

This Divine aspect can now work through you, as you consciously command your persona or ego to step aside. You continue taking action, but now you are free of worries and stress. No longer identified with the doer, you can now just *be*.

# Chapter 7

# The Golden Age of Now

The way to abundance is not through doing, but through *being*. Allowing things and events to unfold is more important than manipulating reality so that it can match our preconceived goals. Once a clear intention as to what we wish to achieve has been set, being open to receive, is more important than a one-sided and imbalanced "going out to get what we want".

In short, a blending of the feminine receptivity with the more male one-pointedness is the way to abundance, not the streotypically male red hot pursuit of our goals. This little change in attitude is an expression of the greater changes which are now occurring.

## The Paradigm of Lack

In the present day and age, we are at a critical juncture in the history of our planet. This is a time of change, a time when a desperately needed shift of consciousness is well under way. Sudden changes have evoked a fear of extinction, which is why today, visions of the final conflagration are immensely popular. Personally, I am not so much concerned about these visions of doom. The fear of the annihilation of all life is more an idea born from the limited view of mankind than an option for Universal Life Force Energy. Actually, the fear of final doom is nothing more than a projection of our own limited beliefs. Since our beliefs are limited, it is easy to project that Life is limited as well.

And yet, although the fear of doom may be insubstantial,

147

we nevertheless live in a time of dramatic change, changes so far reaching, that only a hundred years ago they would have been totally unimaginable. These changes amount to nothing less than an overall shift in paradigm. Shortly, *we all* are going to see life with very different eyes.

Over the last five thousand years, the world has been run on the basis of a few assumed ground rules, such as: God over man, and man over woman. Man is good, woman is evil. Life is struggle, life is lack. So, by looking at history, as it has been taught until now, we can easily see that Life's inherent abundance was not much appreciated over the millenia. For the past five thousand years, it was mostly overlooked, if not repressed, and its presence negated.

Recorded history is a history of strife, conflict and war. We were even taught in history class that "war is the father of all things", presumably because war would force us to invent what is necessary for our own survival. This statement is very revealing, because it shows how impoverishing our whole approach has been. For thousands of years we have stopped living with one another, but have instead fought against one another, each for his or her own survival.

## The Golden Age of Now

All of this is going to change. We are going to experience a re-emergence of abundance consciousness, simply because the old patterns of lack have played themselves out. This shift to a greater openness to Life's inherent abundance will be accompanied by many other shifts, such as: the change from a dominator to a partnership model of society; the change from absolute male control to equality between the sexes; the change from fear and guilt based motivation to motivation based on the creativity and playfulness of Being; the change from exploiting the environment to cooperating with the forces of

Mother Earth; the change from an all-pervasive sense of separation to an all-encompassing experience of non-duality; the change from disdain for the beauty in all of creation to cherishing this beauty from the very bottom of our hearts; the change from feelings of anxiety and insecurity to unconditional love; the change from dichotomy to Unity in true Self.

This may sound too good to be true, but it is actually the only truth—even now, at this very moment. As we have experienced during the practice of the 42-day program to *Core Abundance*, our doubts about such a totally positive and uplifting experience of reality are a direct result of our previous conditioning. It is our conditioning to accept lack as a given, which forces us to continue to experience lack. If you change by letting go of your attachment to your conditioning, you will change your whole experience.

There is actually a precedent from the past, for all the changes which are happening now. There was even a time in history, when Life's inherent abundance was cherished instead of negated. Common to almost all cultures are stories of a Golden Age, when everything was perfect, when there was peace between man and his fellow creatures, and the lifespan of humans was nearly limitless. This Golden age is similar to the Garden of Eden in the *Bible*, or to the first eon as described in many myths of the Hindu and Buddhist tradition. The Golden Age or Paradise represents the garden of boundless Life, out of which man strayed in order to experience the restriction of the material plane—and to grow beyond the need for such experience.

*To live on this Earth of plenty*
*in lands where porpoises guide the ships to harbour*
*and my love dances entranced*
*the snakes of wisdom like bracelets*
*wound around her wrists*
*I relinquish all such thoughts*
*and plunge into heart*
*which is right here right now*

Narayan


In order to understand the myth of a Golden Age and to see how this myth could actually promote the healthier values presented above, we have to look at some curious archeological findings that are rarely mentioned. These findings suggest a previous dramatic shift in mass consciousness which happened gradually between eight thousand and four thousand years ago. It was the exact opposite of the shift we are going to experience now, for the previous shift was from a partnership paradigm to a dominator paradigm, from cooperation to coercion, from equality between the sexes to male domination.

Many clues point to this shift. For example excavations in Eastern and Central Europe reveal that at an earlier period in history, men and women were buried in graves of the same size and with an equal amount of burial objects. All men and women were buried with equal care. Excavations from a later period then revealed a marked difference: the graves of men were now larger. Furthermore, important males were buried together with their wives and slaves (who were killed after the death of their master in order to serve him in the netherworld). There are no indications pointing to similar cruelties in the graves from the earlier periods. Another example is that of fortifications. In excavations from earlier periods, no fortifications were found, whereas excavations from later periods show that fortifications were the norm.

It could be argued that such changes would suggest nothing more but technological progress and by no means a paradigm shift. However, in Crete, in the near East, and in the Indus valley, whole cities without fortifications were excavated. What was found, especially in the cities of the Indus Valley Civilization were sophisticated systems of irrigation, public and private baths, comfortable houses to live in, granaries, sea ports and other highly practical facilities.

It is also interesting to note what was not found, namely buildings that could be considered palaces or temples. No fortifications, no palaces and no temples, but many facilities that made life easier and provided for an ample abundance of fruit, grains, water and comfort—the lands of the Indus Valley Civilization must indeed have been similar to a perfect Garden of Eden where the people lived together in harmony. Even the spiritual aspect of abundance was not lacking, as indicated by clay figurines and seals depicting goddesses and male figures in yoga postures.

In a certain way, our distant past evokes our future, provided we apply the tools necessary to complete the shift in consciousness that has already started. The new innocence we will discover, will be much richer after all the restrictive experiences that we have integrated and transcended over the past five thousand years.

You do not have to wait to make the transition from the old to the new consciousness, you can make the shift now. One major step is to apply yourself with enthusiasm to the 42-day program for dissolving lack, and opening yourself to complete abundance.

In my own life, abundance has been beckoning me for many years. It all started when I became a Reiki master and received guidance to venture into teaching around the world. The abundance I discovered manifested gradually over time, as I learned to trust the inherent goodness and richness of Universal Life Force Energy.

I still work, and sometimes I even choose to work hard, but when I am in touch with the intrinsic awareness of Reiki energy, I experience my work as play. There is ease, flow and grace, and all I am doing is unfolding within Universal Life Force Energy itself.

Only when I am physically exhausted and worn out, do I experience separation from this flow and am thrown back into the old mode of "poor me whose chores and tasks never end". When I am well rested, whatever I am doing feels like a gift that I am given, in order to give back to Life in a process of never ending sharing.

For me, the path of Universal Life Force energy has been one of continuous progress. The many spontaneous initiations into living life fully did not happen over night, but at a regular steady pace. Every person I have ever met has contributed to the process. Every experience I had was valuable, and at one point my beloved teacher clarified this issue of abundance for me once and for all, by giving me a new name. He named me after the Hindu Goddess of Abundance, and said: "I am giving you the name Laxmi, because in this lifetime, you will fulfill all of your desires." I sense that he also realized that my greatest desire, is to dissolve all desires, because my greatest desire is for Freedom. He also stated that he was giving me this new name in order to liberate me from all the old programs of lack, and from the conditioning of my childhood years.

When I look back at my life, I can clearly see that total freedom has always been my intention, and the path that I have chosen to share with others. As I move closer to this state, I see that even freedom is a desire that will eventually melt away, as it is not something that I become, but *THAT* which *I AM*—and to you, dear reader, *THAT* which *you are*.